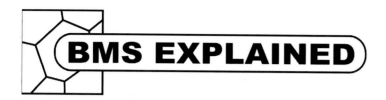

Cellular Pathology

D.J. Cook MPhil BSc FIBMS

Senior Lecturer in Cellular Pathology, University of Portsmouth, School of Pharmacy and Biomedical Science, Portsmouth, UK

Series Editor:

C.J. Pallister PhD MSc FIBMS CBiol MIBiol CHSM

Principal Lecturer in Haematology, Department of Biological and Biomedical Sciences, University of the West of England, Bristol, UK

A member of the Hodder Headline Group
LONDON

First published in Great Britain in 1998 by Butterworth Heinemann.

This impression published in 2003 by
Arnold, a member of the Hodder Headline Group,
338 Euston Road, London NW1 3BH

http://www.arnoldpublishers.com

Distributed in the USA by
Oxford University Press Inc.,
198 Madison Avenue, New York, NY10016
Oxford is a registered trademark of Oxford University Press

Whilst the advice and information in this book are believed to be true and
accurate at the date of going to press, neither the authors nor the publisher
can accept any legal responsibility or liability for any errors or omissions
that may be made. In particular (but without limiting the generality of the
preceding disclaimer) every effort has been made to check drug dosages;
however, it is still possible that errors have been missed. Furthermore,
dosage schedules are constantly being revised and new side-effects
recognized. For these reasons the reader is strongly urged to consult the
drug companies' printed instructions before administering any of the drugs
recommended in this book.

British Library Cataloguing in Publication Data
A catalogue record for this book is available from the British Library

Library of Congress Cataloging-in-Publication Data
A catalog record for this book is available from the Library of Congress

ISBN 0 7506 3111 2

3 4 5 6 7 8 9 10

Printed and bound in Malta by Gutenberg Press

What do you think about this book? Or any other Arnold title?
Please send your comments to feedback.arnold@hodder.co.uk

Contents

Preface

I was pleased when the opportunity to write this book arose. I have often thought that there was not a student oriented book on histological methods. I felt there was a need for a text covering the range of histological topics which was available at a price that undergraduates could afford.

The aim of this book is to be an introductory text for students studying biomedical sciences and it tries to cover the histological techniques used in the diagnosis of disease and in medical research. Many of these students will never become full time histologists and so do not need to know all the details of the techniques. They may, however, need to understand histological technique sufficiently to be able to read scientific papers that use histology, to be able to communicate knowledgeably with histologists in their work. Cost has been kept down by not including all the detailed methods and the omission of experimental detail also allows the book to be shorter.

There are a number of very good laboratory books which are full of useful recipes telling you exactly how to prepare and stain histological sections. For students just beginning their study of histology these recipe books can be quite confusing. The reasons for using a particular technique can be lost in the details of how to actually carry out the stain. This book is intended to be different by being mainly a 'Why?' book rather than a 'How?' book. By that I mean that it attempts to explain the techniques available but does not attempt to give practical details. There are no protocols of methods which can be followed and practical details have been kept to a minimum. I hope to explain the uses of the methods, the advantage of doing one technique rather than another but without giving the full step-by-step instructions.

This does not mean that I think details are unimportant. On the contrary, I think the details of a method are crucial to get a good result. It is just that for most students it is a distraction until they understand the overall concepts. I have referred to books in the recommended reading which are full of excellent recipes and invaluable detail of how to get the best results. I cannot thank the authors of these books enough for the help their books have provided over the years.

I was saddened during the writing of this book to find how many of the books that I rely on have gone out of print. I have deliberately included quite a few of these out-of-print books in the reading lists, in the hope that students will be able to find them in their libraries or obtain them through inter-library loans. The number of currently available books on histological technique is sadly quite small and it seems that in each generation there are only two or three general histological method books in print at any one time. So I urge you to seek out these older books as they are still a mine of useful information.

I have taken the opportunity to extend the range of material covered compared to some laboratory manuals. I have included some techniques which are not currently used. Some are older methods have been superseded by newer, and usually better, techniques but I have included them both for simple historical interest and also because they sometimes have a useful theoretical point . I have also included some research techniques which are only used in relatively few laboratories either because of their interest or because they may become important in the future. I have also included optical illusions in microscopy as it is a particular interest of mine and I think the possibility of microscopists being fooled by what they think they see is not as well known as it should be.

I hope you enjoy the book and find it useful I have certainly enjoyed putting it together.

J. Cook

older method. So this book contains not only the currently important techniques but also some less popular ones.

Preparing tissues alters them

All the techniques used in histological preparation have their own particular problems and all produce significant changes in the tissues. These changes in the tissues are grouped together as **artefacts**. Artefacts are changes in the tissue brought about by the techniques used, they are errors introduced during the processing of tissues. The artefacts that can be produced are as many and as varied as the techniques which produce them. It would take several pages just to list all the artefacts that can occur but artefacts can be grouped into three major types. Within each type there will be a variety of causes and a range of individual errors but if we can understand the types of errors it often helps us to recognize the errors and sometimes helps us to know how to avoid them.

> The term artefacts can also be spelt artifacts. They are both pronounced the same but I prefer the 'e' since it comes from the Latin *arte* (by art) but others disagree.
>
> The most bizarre artefact I've seen was a complete small spider in a stained section. During the drying of the section a student had used a hotplate and put the section face up on the hotplate. A spider must have fallen on it, was killed and dried down. The student never noticed, stained the section and then, when it was being examined under the microscope, there in the middle of the kidney was a spider.

Materials can be lost during section preparation

The loss of material from the tissue is one of the commonest types of artefact. Sometimes it is not a disaster if materials are lost, provided the important materials, and in particular the substance we are looking for, are retained.

If we take paraffin wax processed tissues as an example, the materials that are lost from the tissues include:

- All the small water soluble molecules. These tend to be lost when we attempt to preserve the tissue by immersing it in a fixative. The materials lost include simple sugars (glucose, fructose etc.), ions (sodium, potassium, chlorides, sulphates, phosphates etc.), vitamins (thiamine, riboflavin etc.), cofactors (ADP, NAD etc.) and many others.
- All the lipids and lipid soluble materials that are extracted by the alcohols, clearing agents and hot waxes used in preparing wax sections. This means that all the membrane lipids, steroid hormones and fat soluble vitamins are lost as well as the simple adipose fats.

So it is no use preparing a paraffin wax section to try and identify where the NAD was located within a cell because it will all have disappeared. In paraffin wax section just about the only things that are retained are the proteins, some nucleic acids and a few other molecules. What is perhaps more surprising is how much information about tissue structure and function can be learnt from such a depleted material.

Materials can be gained during section preparation

This usually involves chemical additions to the structures. Any material prepared using aldehydes as preservatives will have extra aldehydes that were not there in life. Aldehydes form addition compounds (see Chapter 2) with at least some of the amine groups in proteins. If the preservation is done with mercury compounds instead of aldehydes then there will be a black deposit of mercury within the tissues that was not there before the fixative was added.

These chemical additions are an inherent part of the technique but there are also additions that can be less predictable. For example, during the handling of the tissues in the laboratory the blocks may be placed on filter paper or handled with rubber gloves. Fibres from the paper or glove powder from the gloves may be accidentally transferred to the specimen and appear in the final preparation. These contaminants are artefacts since they were not there in the living body.

Materials and structures can be altered or distorted during section preparation

The most common distortion is that tissues shrink during processing. Shrinkage in itself is not a serious problem provided everything alters to the same extent. As long as the shrinkage is regular then we can compare tissues with each other knowing that they will have been affected to the same degree. Unfortunately shrinkage is often irregular. Some materials shrink more than others and give a false impression. Take bone as an example. Bone consists of a very hard matrix containing a few scattered cells called osteocytes which lie in little spaces in the bone called lacunae. In life the whole of the lacunae are filled by the cytoplasm of the osteocytes. But during sectioning the soft tissue of the osteocyte shrinks much more than the hard matrix. As a result, in many sections of bone the osteocytes appear shrunken and a gap appears around the cells. This gap is an artefact of the processing.

All sections have some artefacts

Whenever a section is seen there will be artefacts and the recognition of these is an important part of histology. It is also important to be able to avoid certain artefacts and so histologists need a range of methods which have different properties so they can always manage to get a section which will show them what is needed. It may have other artefacts but the section will avoid the specific artefacts that would make it useless for a particular purpose. By carefully selecting a method certain artefacts can be avoided but all sections have some artefacts. So wax sections do not contain lipids but they do not have any ice crystal damage. Frozen sections retain the lipids but may show ice crystal damage. You must choose your method to suit your requirements.

Fortunately histological workers over the history of the subject have been very clever in approaching the problems in different ways and so most of what we now acknowledge as the structure of cells and tissues stands on a very firm base. But whenever the boundaries of a technique are extended it is always correct to ask 'is this real or is this just the result of what has been done to the tissues?'.

Histology is constantly evolving and changing

The preparation of tissues has constantly been improving and it seems likely that it will continue to improve in future. The earliest microscopists simply used whole mounts of small specimens with little or no use of dyeing. The earliest sections used free hand-sectioning but this gives only poor results and it was the introduction of the technique of embedding tissues in a solid medium and the use of dyes to enhance contrast and visibility which made histology into an accurate and reliable method.

The embedding techniques have been many and varied. Using these differing techniques much of the tissue structure still remains very similar. The appearances do change slightly, but by comparing techniques it is possible to determine the structures of the tissues as they would be inside the living animal or human. We can therefore also state with confidence that one technique will cause shrinkage, another will destroy some tissue components and yet another may alter the chemical nature of the tissues. Whenever a piece of tissue is to be investigated the choice of the preparative technique will impose its own limitations and advantages. A single technique is never the best for every possible situation. You must know what you want to see and then choose the appropriate method. So in this book there will be a description of several alternative techniques and a comparison of their advantages and problems.

Demonstration techniques are now much more selective and specific

One of the major advances has been the improvement of demonstration methods. In the earliest years of micro-technique the only methods available to demonstrate structure was to use the few natural dyes that were available. These were often unreliable and the demonstrations were poor and did not keep well. The phenomenal increase in the number of dyes available following the synthesis of dyes (particularly from coal tar) made it possible to produce more selective methods and brighter colours. The use of many of these techniques is still an important part of micro-technique today. The development of the use of antibodies and histochemical techniques has allowed even more precision and it is

Histology is one area of science where there is a great deal of manual skill needed as well as scientific knowledge. The ability to cut sections is certainly crucial to obtaining acceptable results and a good microtomist needs a long apprenticeship. Staining requires skills in differentiation to get the optimal contrast in specimens. This has led to a certain amount of mystique in histology and the assertion that histology is more of an art than a science.

The results of histology are slides and these can certainly be aesthetically pleasing in an abstract way but they are always based on scientific principles. Histologists do not actually create the results, they just bring out what is present in the tissues. Histochemistry in particularly is as pure a science as any other science.

The other assertion is that histology is getting left behind. This again is not true. Histology may be involved with dyeing but it is not a dying art!

now possible to identify and localize individual molecules and chemicals rather than just the vague staining of 'proteins'. Now there is a rapidly increasing use of nucleic acid techniques that have unprecedented accuracy and can identify the actual genes and mutations of genes which are associated with many diseases. Where this will lead in the future is not absolutely clear but histological micro-technique is certainly not a dead-end with no significant further developments but a lively and growing scientific discipline.

Histology is likely to change dramatically in future

Histological techniques have not altered as much in the past century as those of other scientific disciplines such as biochemistry. A histologist from the late 19th century would probably adjust to working in a modern laboratory with little difficulty. He might need a little retraining in the advances that have taken place but at least he would understand the general concepts. Biochemistry, on the other hand, has changed dramatically and a 19th century biochemist would not recognize most of the instruments and techniques that are now routine. My feelings are that histological micro-technique will undergo a similar change in the coming years. It will be more important to understand the concepts behind the methods than to know the best recipe for a stain since many of the current techniques will become obsolete and will be replaced. Only the underlying principles are likely to remain the same and will be equally important in 50 years' time as they will be in 5 years' time.

This book, unlike the majority of textbooks on histological technique, is not a practical book full of recipes and methods, but aims to be an introduction to the concepts of tissue preparation. This does not mean that I think the detail of the techniques is unimportant. I believe that the details and tips present in the laboratory recipe books are often quite fascinating in themselves and are also essential to anyone intending to work in a histological laboratory or use histology in a regular and practical way. The detail is always important when you come to actually prepare a tissue section, but when you are just beginning to learn about the subject the detail may get in the way of a deeper understanding. When you want to do histology then you will need a laboratory manual but I hope that having read this book first you will be able to follow the method with understanding and not just an unthinking adherence to the recipe.

This book is also intended for people who are not themselves intending to become histologists but who will be working alongside histologists, who will need to talk to histologists and perhaps even make use of histology but without needing to do all the preparation themselves. You may not need to know the minute to minute steps in preparing tissues, but if you are going to understand histology

Histology is still one of the most important research methods. A quick look in any major biomedical or biological journal will show that more than half of the papers will include some histological aspect. Histology can appeal to humans in a way that most scientific disciplines do not. Histology is an essentially visual science and human beings are highly visual, with the amount of information received and understood through vision being greater than all the other senses combined. The display of a good histological preparation always appeals both aesthetically and intellectually since it is possible to see for oneself. No amount of tables or graphs can have quite the same impact as a good section.

and histologists then you need to understand their problems and their language.

Like all scientific disciplines, histology is absolutely enthralling to its disciples but can often seem boring and routine to non-histologists. I hope to try and bridge the gap between these extremes and show the fascination but without the tedious detail, to show the scope that histology can cover. And if, in the process, I can make you think that histological methodology is worthwhile learning then I will feel that the book has succeeded.

Suggested further reading

Wallington, E.A. (1979). Artifacts in tissue sections. *Medical Laboratory Sciences* **36**, 3–61.

Self-assessment questions

1. Outline what is meant by an artefact.
2. List the major types of artefact and give one example of each type.
3. Two sections are prepared by different methods to show the location of glycogen. The first section shows glycogen in hepatocytes (liver cells) evenly spread throughout the cells. The second shows glycogen present in the same cells but concentrated at one end of the cell.
   Can we conclude that hepatocytes contain glycogen?
   Can we conclude that glycogen is evenly spread in the hepatocytes?
4. Why is there no single method of tissue preparation that everyone agrees is the best?

Key Concepts and Facts

- Histology is the study of tissue structure.

- Cellular pathology is the study of diseases in tissues.

- Tissues need to be sectioned and stained to allow their structure to be seen.

- All preparation alters the tissue and these alterations are called artefacts.

- Artefacts can be losses of material, the addition of material or distortion of tissue structures.

Chapter 2
Fixation and fixatives

Learning objectives

After studying this chapter you should confidently be able to:

Describe why tissue removed from the body will change.

Describe how fixatives stop post-mortem changes.

List the properties of a perfect fixative.

Discuss how different fixatives have special properties and uses in histology.

Describe how simple fixatives can be used in combination to improve preservation.

Human cells and tissues in the body can remain alive because they are connected to the bloodstream which provides them with the oxygen and nutrients they need and also removes the toxic waste products of metabolism. If the blood circulation stops, or if the tissues are removed from the body during an operation, then the cells will be cut off from this essential life-support system. If cells are deprived of oxygen for long enough then they will die. In histology we want to see the cells looking exactly the same as they were in the living body so the tissue must be stabilized as quickly as possible after the cells lose the blood circulation. This is done by fixation.

Types of tissue change

The way in which tissues change can vary depending on the organ involved but we can identify three types of change which occur in all tissues.

- **The cells do not die instantly when the blood circulation stops but remain alive by drawing on their energy supplies and respiring anaerobically.** This is a useful response since cells often get temporarily cut off from circulating blood, for example lying for a long time on your arm in bed restricts the blood flow. When you move and allow the blood to recirculate into the area it results in 'pins and needles' due to the accumula-

---

The ability of cells to survive away from the body depends on their individual energy stores. Some cells have large stores of glycogen, examples include skin, muscle and heart tissue. Other cells have very little in the way of stored energy and are totally dependent on a regular supply of glucose, e.g. the neurones in the brain. Muscle and skin can therefore survive using their own supplies for considerable lengths of time, probably in excess of 20 minutes, but the brain will be permanently damaged in less than 2 minutes if totally deprived of a blood supply. So it is safe to put a tourniquet around an arm or a leg to arrest bleeding but it is not safe to put a tourniquet around the neck for even a few seconds.

tion of waste products including lactic acid and carbon dioxide, both of which are acidic. If the cell was left without a blood supply for many minutes the cells would die; this is the cause of bedsores. The affected cells would then be different to the state they were in before the blood supply ceased. They would have exhausted their store of glycogen and would be more acidic than normal tissues due to the lactic acid and carbon dioxide. Both of these can result in visible changes in the cell.

- **When the cells die they begin to break down.** The most important part of this breakdown occurs when the lysosomes release their enzymes into the cell cytoplasm. These enzymes include proteases which destroy proteins, nucleases which destroy nucleic acids and lipases which destroy lipids. This will eventually result in the complete disintegration of the cell and its contents. This process of self-digestion is called **autolysis.**
- **If bacteria or fungal spores alight on tissues,** particularly dead tissues, then **they can begin to grow** and this will result in microbial spoilage or **putrefaction** and this will drastically alter the structure of the tissues.

Putrefaction is not the most important change in histology

Collectively these changes are sometimes referred to as post-mortem changes. It is the last form of tissue decay, putrefaction, that tends to be identified by most people as the most important form of change in pieces of tissue, but in histological terms this is a slow and therefore less important form of change than autolysis and abnormal metabolism.

Putrefaction is important in dealing with meat in everyday life since bacterial contamination can lead to food poisoning. Fortunately for butchers the process is very slow so that, provided the meat is kept cool, it will not spoil by bacterial growth.

Most tissues removed from the body are quite sterile and need to be contaminated from the air before bacterial growth can even start. Autolysis is more rapid but is not a disadvantage for culinary meat, indeed it is an advantage since it helps to tenderize the meat and improve the flavour. The traditional 'hanging' of meat for several days makes use of autolysis to improve its eating qualities.

The different types and rates of change allow pathologists to estimate how long a body has been dead and this can be important in forensic pathology.

Fixation

Fixation is an attempt to preserve the tissues in a life-like condition. Fixation must stop abnormal enzyme activity and metabolism, in other words kill the cells, and it must stop autolysis by inactivating the lysosomal enzymes. Most fixatives are therefore enzyme poisons. Killing enzymes will also stop bacterial and fungal growth and so prevent putrefactive changes.

Fixation is usually achieved by immersing the tissues in a chemical solution hence it is referred to as chemical fixation but it can also be achieved by heat. Bacteriologists have traditionally fixed their bacterial smears by passing them through a Bunsen flame. High temperatures destroy enzyme activity and so act as a form of fixation. This is not common in histology since it is difficult to control but it has been used for rapid fixation or in some histochemical investigations where the use of chemical solutions would interfere with the chemical reactions. Microwave ovens have made this form of fixation easier to apply and control and are

The process of fixation is not new. Preservation of meat for cooking is an old technology. In food preservation the processes can be slowed by removing the water. In the absence of water enzymes cannot act, metabolism is stopped and bacterial growth is greatly retarded.

Water can be removed by simple drying in air, or by using salt to extract the water. Both will work with human tissue as well as with meat for food. The process is called mummification after the Egyptian mummies which were dried using salts and preserved using oils and resins. The tissue is, however, desiccated and shrunken, making mummification a poor method of preservation for histology.

Although simple drying of tissues is not a good method by modern standards some tissue structures can still be seen and identified in mummies over 5000 years old.

probably the best way to heat-fix tissues, and microwave fixation is becoming increasingly popular.

There are many chemicals that act as enzyme poisons but only a few are useful as histological fixatives. No fixative can perfectly preserve any tissues exactly the way it was in life but some fixatives can give very good histological results for certain restricted purposes.

A perfect fixative needs several properties

Before considering some common fixatives it is useful to identify the properties which we would like to see in a perfect fixative.

A perfect fixative should:

- Penetrate tissues quickly and evenly; this makes all parts of the tissues look the same. If penetration is uneven then the edges of the tissue will look quite different to the centre of the specimen.
- Kill cells quickly and evenly; the killing stops abnormal metabolism.
- Prevent autolysis.
- Prevent putrefaction.
- Not add any extraneous material to the tissue.
- Not swell or shrink the tissue.
- Prepare the tissue for later treatments such as staining and should not prevent any later investigation that might be needed.
- Prevent desiccation and drying of tissue which would cause shrinkage and distortion.
- Be safe to use (non-toxic, non-flammable).
- Be reasonably priced.
- Be convenient to use (shelf-life, storage etc.).

The first seven properties are related to how the fixative affects the tissues whilst the last three are related to practical use of the fixative in the laboratory.

No reagent has all of these properties and fixation is always a compromise and is always less than perfect.

Fixatives

The following are a few of the commoner fixatives that are used for preserving tissues.

Formaldehyde (HCHO)

This is a pungent toxic gas which is soluble in water. It is usually sold as a 37–40% solution of formaldehyde in water, when it is called **formalin** (in the UK formalin is a general term but in some countries it is a trade mark). It is the most widely used fixative for routine light microscopy sections when it is used as a 4% solution of formaldehyde. Note that 4% formaldehyde is made by diluting the formalin solution (i.e. 40% formaldehyde) using one part of the formalin with nine parts of water (a one in 10 dilution) and it is often called 10% formalin. The terms formalin and formaldehyde are both still in common use but the concentrations are quite different. So 10% formalin is exactly the same strength as 4% formaldehyde. The use of formaldehyde concentrations rather than formalin concentrations is the preferred method.

Formaldehyde is a very reactive chemical and undergoes several changes in storage. Formalin solutions are usually impure and contain a number of contaminants, some added by the manufacturer and others formed during storage.

In aqueous solution formaldehyde reacts with water forming methylene glycol:

$$HCHO + H_2O \rightarrow CH_2(OH)_2$$

Formic acid (methanoic acid) can be formed by oxidation of formaldehyde by the oxygen in air:

$$2\,HCHO + O_2 \rightarrow 2\,HCOOH$$

and also by the Canizzaro reaction:

$$2\,HCHO + H_2O \rightarrow HCOOH + CH_3OH$$

Methanol is also formed in this reaction. Methanol is deliberately added to formalin solutions by the manufacturers, partly to inhibit this Canizzaro reaction and also to prevent polymerization. Methyl methanoate can also be formed by esterification of the methanol and methanoic acid.

Finally, formaldehyde polymerizes to form 'paraformaldehyde':

$$n\,HCHO \leftrightarrow HO(CH_2)_n H + (n-1)\,H_2O$$

This occurs especially in the cold conditions found in most chemical stores.

The paraformaldehyde does not harm the fixative except by reducing the formaldehyde concentration. Provided this is adjusted to take account of the loss the final solution will still fix tissues very well. If the polymer formed is a short chain of less than eight formaldehyde molecules then the paraformaldehyde is still soluble and will not be noticed, but if the chains are longer than eight carbons then it precipitates as a white powder. The paraformaldehyde will depolymerize if warmed or diluted. Depolymerization is more rapid if the solution is around neutral pH.

Thus the commercial formalin solutions are really quite impure. The most important contaminant is the methanoic acid which will affect the pH and the fixing properties. Acid formalin will, for example, produce a brown deposit around degenerating blood cells. This is an artefact and is therefore a nuisance although it can be removed by dissolving in alcoholic picric acid. To prevent this

The acidity of formalin solutions led some laboratories to try and combat the build-up of acidity by adding calcium carbonate chips to the stock formalin bottles. The acid would then be neutralized because as the acid was formed it would react with the carbonate forming calcium methanoate (formate). Although this will work it also releases carbon dioxide. If the bottle is firmly capped the build-up of pressure can cause the bottle to explode, and if the bottle is not firmly capped then not only can the carbon dioxide escape but also the formaldehyde vapours which are toxic and irritant. Both situations are to be avoided.

Formaldehyde is a very dangerous chemical and should be handled carefully. Contact with the skin can result in an allergic reaction due to the formalin attacking skin proteins and modifying their structure sufficiently to make the body identify them as foreign. The immune system will then start attacking these proteins and this results in severe disease.

Always use protective gloves and clothing when dealing with formaldehyde.

Formaldehyde is also a respiratory poison and must only be used in a well-ventilated area. The ventilation must carry the fumes **away** from the face, so downward or backward ventilating systems are needed. Upward ventilation can actually pull the vapour towards the mouth and nose.

occurring only neutral formaldehyde solutions should be used. Simple neutralizing of the acid with alkali or calcium carbonate are less satisfactory than buffering (usually with a phosphate buffer) and most laboratories normally use buffered formaldehyde as their routine fixative.

If greater purity is needed, as it often is for critical applications such as electron microscopy, then it is better not to use commercial formalin solutions. Instead formaldehyde can be generated by depolymerizing paraformaldehyde. The paraformaldehyde is un-adulterated and not contaminated in the same way as the commercial formalin solutions and is more reliable and purer.

Fixation properties

Formaldehyde in solution is almost entirely in the hydrated form of methylene glycol and it is the methylene glycol that acts as the fixative. The glycol adds on to proteins forming single and double additions:

$$CH_2(OH)_2 + R\text{-}NH_2 \leftrightarrow R\text{-}NHCH_2OH + H_2O$$

$$R\text{-}NHCH_2OH + R_2\text{-}NH_2 \rightarrow R\text{-}NHCH_2HNR_2 + H_2O$$

Single additions are easily reversed by washing in water for a few hours. Double reactions are more stable and produce methylene bridges.

These reactions occur slowly over a period of days so formaldehyde is a slow-acting fixative and full fixation takes about a week though adequate fixation occurs in 12–24 h.

As well as its main fixative properties, formaldehyde has several other advantages as a routine fixative. The effect of formaldehyde on tissues is to cause them to swell slightly, and this means the organs remain soft and pliable. This soft fixation is good for dissection and for trimming of tissues into blocks for processing. Many other fixatives harden the tissue, making trimming and dissection difficult or impossible. The tissue does, however, harden during processing so the final paraffin block is very hard.

It is a very tolerant and forgiving fixative. Tissues cannot be overfixed and can be stored in formalin for many years. Many other fixatives can overfix the tissue and formaldehyde is often used to store tissues originally fixed in such fixatives.

Most fixatives alter the colour of tissues, often turning them a dull greyish colour. Formaldehyde is the only fixative that allows natural colour to be restored and so it is the basis of all museum fixatives.

Formaldehyde is not perfect; it has its drawbacks. Cytoplasmic staining is duller after simple formaldehyde fixation than it is after many other fixatives. Formaldehyde is also toxic and causes formalin dermatitis and is a cancer suspect agent.

Glutaraldehyde

Glutaraldehyde is a bifunctional aldehyde which reacts more quickly than formaldehyde (it binds to 90% of NH_2 groups in 2 h; HCHO binds to only 70% of such groups in 7 days). It polymerizes very easily and glutaraldehyde solutions should be depolymerized before use.

It is difficult to remove the glutaraldehyde from tissue and this makes histochemistry difficult – in particular many aldehydes remain active since each molecule has two aldehyde groups and often only one is actually bound to the tissues and the second group therefore remains active. The extra aldehydes prevent glutaraldehyde being a useful fixative when the PAS reaction and other aldehyde-detecting reagents are being used. It inactivates all enzymes, so totally preventing enzyme histochemistry. It also binds and masks many antigens, making immunotechniques difficult or even impossible.

Glutaraldehyde fixation gives excellent morphology but staining with acidic dyes is depressed. Like formaldehyde it is very dangerous if inhaled or brought in contact with the skin. Glutaraldehyde is widely used in electron microscopy.

Mercuric chloride

Mercuric chloride is a white crystalline solid soluble to about 7% in water. It is highly toxic as a cumulative poison, so small doses over a long period can gradually build up to a toxic dose.

It fixes tissues by attaching to SH groups in proteins and it crosslinks them forming a coarse coagulum of protein. Coagulating fixatives such as mercuric chloride leave relatively large fluid-filled spaces within the protein and allow rapid penetration of reagents into the tissues through these channels. Staining is not depressed since mercuric chloride does not block the NH_2 groups in the same way as the aldehyde fixatives and the cytoplasm stains brightly with acid dyes. The coagulation, however, leaves the tissue excessively hard and shrinks the tissue considerably. For this reason it is never used alone but only in association with other softer fixatives.

Mercuric chloride leaves a black precipitate (mercury pigment) in tissues which interferes with the appearance and needs to be removed. The pigment is easily removed with iodine, which converts it to mercuric iodide, followed by sodium thiosulphate (often referred to as 'hypo') which removes the mercuric iodide.

Mercuric chloride is less used than previously because of its cost, toxicity and the difficulty of disposing of the waste fixative.

Mercuric chloride was previously called 'corrosive sublimate'. The 'corrosive' refers to the fact that it attacks virtually all metals (including gold). So care is needed when using mercuric chloride as it will corrode jewellery (including wedding rings), scalpels and metal forceps. It will corrode metal piping, so prolonged disposal down laboratory sinks has been known to rot metal waste pipes and resulted in flooding of some labs.

Mercury and its compounds should not in any case be disposed of down the sink as it is toxic to the sewage bacteria and will contaminate the effluent from sewage works.

Osmium tetroxide

Osmium tetroxide is very expensive (up to £80,000 per kilogram) so it is usually restricted to fixing very small pieces of tissue. It is a powerful oxidizing agent and adds on to double bonds and in so doing it blackens them. Since most lipids contain double bonds it fixes lipids and it is the only fixative that really does so. For this reason it is widely used to fix the lipid membranes in electron microscopy.

Fixation in osmium tetroxide makes proteins lose their acidophilia. It is volatile and can react with the cornea, resulting in blindness. It must be handled only in fume cupboards.

It is widely used in electron microscopy as a fixative and stain for membranes but very rarely used as a light microscopy fixative.

Acetic acid (ethanoic acid)

Although the correct chemical name is ethanoic acid this is rarely heard in histology laboratories and the older, less systematic name, of acetic acid is universally used. Unlike all the preceding fixatives acetic acid is a non-additive fixative and does not bind to any chemical groups in the tissues. It has its main effect by denaturing nucleic acids by pH effects. It does not fix proteins and causes them to swell (especially collagen), and it effectively destroys mitochondrial staining.

Acetic acid is widely used to improve nuclear staining since it preserves DNA very well without blocking any dye binding sites. The poor cytoplasmic staining from the loss of protein is an advantage in some types of work, e.g. chromosome studies where poor cytoplasmic preservation leaves the chromosomes more easily observed against a clear background. If a good cytoplasmic fixation is achieved the cytoplasm will stain strongly and this will obscure the fine chromosome structure.

Acetic acid has often been included in fixative mixtures to combat the shrinkage of other fixatives.

Alcohols (methanol, ethanol, propanol, butanol etc.)

These are also non-additive fixatives which denature proteins and nucleic acids by removing their bound water and replacing it with the alcohol. This alters the shape of molecules (tertiary structure) without altering the reactive groups. So alcohols preserve the chemical reactivity of many cellular materials and are popular in histochemical investigations.

The tissues do shrink considerably and may become overhard and brittle if long alcohol fixation is used. Alcohol is therefore less commonly used for fixing blocks of tissue but is common for fixing smears or fresh sections (cryostat sections; see Chapter 5) where it is less of a problem if the cells become brittle as no further sectioning is needed.

Alcoholic fixation is probably more widespread than is acknowledged because a poorly fixed specimen is often processed unknowingly. The alcohol used in processing then acts as the fixative for any unfixed parts of the block.

The use of alcohol and acetic acid has a long history in food preservation. Peaches in brandy and pickled onions are both highly regarded delicacies by many people.

Alcohol is also one of the oldest embalming techniques. Following his death at the battle of Trafalgar, Nelson's body was placed in a barrel of brandy to preserve it during the journey back to Britain.

Many other chemicals have fixative properties, and fixatives in reasonably common use include picric acid, potassium dichromate and chromic acid. They all have some useful characteristics but their properties will not be dealt with in detail here.

Practical fixative solutions

Although the simple fixatives are the major component of most practical fixative solutions they are rarely used as pure solutions and are usually made up with other compounds. These other components are often very important to the final result but are not directly involved in the fixation. They are used to control the environment around and within the tissues whilst fixation occurs.

The various types of additive can be grouped into three classes:

- **To control tonicity (osmotic pressure).** Living cells are osmotic systems and will shrink in hypertonic solutions (high salt concentration) and swell and even burst in hypotonic solutions (pure water or low salt concentration). Blood plasma and cell cytoplasm has a tonicity of about 340 mOsm and this is said to be isotonic. The final tonicity of many practical fixatives is made hypertonic at around 400–450 mOsm. This is to ensure that even when the fixative is removed during the fixation process the residual solution is still at least isotonic and will not cause cellular lysis due to osmotic imbalance. If the fluid became hypotonic before fixation was achieved the cells might absorb water by osmosis, resulting in swelling and eventual lysis.

- **To control pH.** The use of buffers is preferred. Many buffers can be used, including phosphate, Tris and cacodylates. The choice of buffer is controlled by other components. Phosphate buffers will precipitate if calcium or magnesium ions are added whilst Tris and barbiturate buffers will react with aldehyde fixatives.

- **Other materials for specific reasons.** For example, calcium is sometimes added to help preserve phospholipids, ammonium bromide is said to enhance the fixation of nervous tissue (particularly neuroglia), and detergents are used to remove membrane lipids and aid penetration of the fixative and other reagents such as lectins.

The physical conditions also play a major role so the temperature, volume and duration of fixation can also be critical.

Short fixation is common in histochemistry especially when fixing frozen sections (2 min at 4°C, for example). Prolonged fixation in most reagents will result in overfixation and the tissue may become unusable. Even formaldehyde, which is often used for long-term storage of specimens, does slowly alter the tissue, e.g. the ability of the tissue to stain with acid dyes becomes diminished.

The volume of fixative should be very large compared to the volume of tissue (20 times is a safe margin) since the fixative gets

Unfortunately fixation is often left to people who aren't histologists. These include operating theatre staff who all too often mistakenly believe that the most important form of tissue breakdown is bacterial decay and so put tissues into antiseptics or disinfectants. These will certainly kill bacteria but they do little else to preserve the tissues. Whenever possible either do the fixation yourself or make sure the person who does it understands what is needed, otherwise poor fixation and poor preservation will be the result.

I have personally received specimens from operating theatres in antiseptic solutions such as Savlon with dreadful results and even once in a Domestos solution which certainly killed the germs but did little to enhance the tissue preservation. I also received one specimen from a general dental practitioner in gin. This gave adequate preservation but I would not recommend it as a general fixative.

depleted or diluted by the tissue. This is often overlooked with very large specimens which are crammed into too small a container that is then topped up with fixative. A large ovarian cyst (whose total volume may be a litre or more) may arrive in the laboratory with less than 100 ml of fixative poured over it.

If the specimen is large and penetration is likely to be poor then either the fixative should be perfused into the blood vessels and pumped through the vascular channels so that it reaches all the parts of the tissue very quickly or the block should be cut into pieces small enough for diffusion of the fixative to reach all parts in a reasonable time.

Compound fixatives

Since every simple fixative has deficiencies many people have tried to improve fixation by using more than one fixative in a solution. The intention is to use one fixative's good properties to counteract the bad properties of the other components.

For example, Zenker's fixative is based on mercuric chloride but has acetic acid and potassium dichromate added to modify the results. Mercuric chloride was chosen to give good cytoplasmic staining but it suffers from being a very harsh fixative, causing excessive hardening and shrinkage if used alone. Although a good protein fixative it is less good with nucleic acids and lipids. Acetic acid causes swelling which counteracts the shrinkage, it gives a softer fixation, ameliorating the hard fixation of the mercuric chloride, and finally it fixes nucleic acid very well. Unfortunately it does not fix lipids at all. Potassium dichromate preserves some lipids especially phospholipids of membranes. It improves cytoplasmic staining but it may dissolve nucleic acids (however, acetic acid counteracts this effect). The overall result is a good general fixation and Zenker has become a widely accepted fixative.

In formulating a compound fixative some provisos should be noted. The fixatives chosen may add their own disadvantages without counteracting the bad points of the other fixatives. This summation of bad points can result in worse fixation than if only one fixative was used.

Mixing fixatives of different penetrating power may result in very uneven fixation with only the outer part of the tissue being fixed in the full mixture. The slowest penetrating fixative may lag so far behind the other fixatives that the inner parts are fixed only by the faster diffusing components.

It can also cause problems if the component chemicals can react with each other. Aldehydes are reducing agents whilst osmium tetroxide is an oxidizing agent, so any solution containing both will rapidly deteriorate.

Finally, the use of several component fixatives means that it becomes difficult to predict all the chemical reactions occurring during fixation, so compound fixatives are not usually the best fixatives for critical histochemistry.

Although compound fixatives can be an improvement on simple fixatives they still cannot be ideal for every purpose and each is usually designed for different and specific purposes, for example:

- **Micro-anatomical** fixatives (Zenker, SUSA) are excellent for preserving general tissue structure and fixing larger blocks evenly, but will be less good for cytological detail.
- **Cytological** fixatives are often good at preserving fine cytological detail in small blocks, but are less useful for giving even fixation if the blocks are larger. Within the cytological fixatives there is further specialization since nucleic acids and cytoplasm are very different materials.

Nuclear fixatives (Carnoy, Flemming with acetic acid) will preserve nuclei very well whilst **cytoplasmic fixatives** (Helly, Flemming without acetic acid) are preferred for cytoplasmic detail.

Fixation is usually associated with science but Damien Hirst achieved notoriety by using animals in formaldehyde as examples of modern art. He exhibited a sheep in formaldehyde titled 'Away from the Flock' at the Serpentine Gallery in 1994 and it was reputedly sold for £25,000. The mummified remains of the pharaohs have been icons of history for generations and the embalmed body of Lenin is an important tourist attraction in Moscow. So preservation is also important outside the laboratory.

Post-fixation

This is a similar concept to compound fixatives with the benefits of one fixative being added to those of another but the fixatives are used sequentially rather than as a single solution. The primary fixative is almost always an aldehyde but the secondary fixative varies, with post-chroming (potassium dichromate), post-subliming (mercuric chloride) and post-osmicating (osmium tetroxide) all having their place.

Importance of correct fixation

When choosing a fixative it is important to get it right. Properly fixed tissues are easier to prepare and the final results are better. Poor or inappropriate fixation makes later processing and staining more difficult and may make certain investigations impossible. So before fixing tissues, and indeed before starting to remove them from the body, the final purpose of the sections must be considered and the fixation chosen to match the requirements of the technique. Trying to match a staining technique to an inappropriately fixed tissue always gives inferior results.

Suggested further reading

Hopwood, D. (1996). Fixation and fixatives, in *Theory and Practice of Histological Techniques* (eds J.D. Bancroft and A. Stevens). Edinburgh: Churchill Livingstone.

Kiernan, J.A. (1990). *Histological and Histochemical Methods.* Oxford: Pergamon.

Self-assessment questions

1. In what ways will tissue removed from the body change with time?
2. How can post-mortem changes be prevented?
3. List the properties of a good fixative.
4. Dettol will kill bacteria including those that cause putrefaction. Will Dettol be a good fixative?
5. Schiff's reagent is used to detect naturally occurring aldehydes in tissues. It can be used easily on formaldehyde fixed tissues but not on glutaraldehyde fixed tissues.
   Why is there this difference?
6. Why should all fixatives be handled and treated carefully?

Key Concepts and Facts

Tissue Degeneration
- Tissues can degenerate by three mechanisms.
- Putrefaction is destruction by micro-organisms.
- Autolysis is degeneration by lysosomal enzymes.
- Abnormal metabolism occurs in isolated tissues.

Fixation
- Fixation is the attempt to stop tissue degenerating and preserve it in a life-like condition.
- Fixatives are usually enzyme poisons.
- All fixatives have drawbacks and there is no single perfect fixative.
- Fixatives can be used in combination to improve preservation.
- Fixative solutions must be mixed with salts and buffers to control osmotic pressure and pH.
- The fixative should be chosen to match the investigation.
- Good fixation is essential for good sections.

Chapter 3
Processing and microtomy

Learning objectives

After studying this chapter you should confidently be able to:

Describe why tissue needs support during sectioning.

Describe how tissues can be impregnated with wax using inter-mediate reagents.

Name several common and useful dehydrating and clearing agents.

Describe the preparation of mineralized tissues for sectioning.

Outline the characteristics of a microtome and microtome knives.

Even fixed human tissues are generally quite soft and need extra support to allow thin sections to be cut. Sections are usually cut between 3 and 6 μm thick and the easiest way to prepare sections of this thickness is to use a hard embedding medium to support the cells and to hold the tissue firmly. **Processing** is the method by which tissues are converted into a block for **microtomy**.

Paraffin wax impregnation

The commonest embedding medium in routine histology is paraffin wax. Although called a wax the materials are actually long-chain paraffin hydrocarbons and are similar to the materials used to make candles. Paraffin wax is molten at above 60°C but is solid at room temperature and has a hardness similar to the tissues once they have been impregnated. However, the specimen cannot be simply immersed in the wax since wax and water are immiscible and simply putting the tissue in molten wax will only result in the tissue being coated in wax (see Box). The water in the tissues is instead replaced by wax so that the support runs completely through the tissues and supports them internally as well as externally (wax impregnation). The replacement of the tissue water with wax involves several steps and is generally called processing. One or more intermediate processing reagents are

Originally the support for tissues was much less intimate and did not penetrate into the tissue but simply surrounded it. Botanists still often support stems and leaves for cutting by wrapping them in elder pith to make a more rigid structure. This is less easy to do with animal tissues which are much more irregular in shape and are less intrinsically rigid than plant tissues. Histologists therefore used wax. The tissues were dipped in molten wax that moulded itself to the irregular shape of the tissue and helped support it. This was still not successful and it was not until the wax was permeated into the tissue as well as around it that effective sectioning was possible.

needed to remove the water, replace it with a reagent miscible with wax and then finally impregnate with the wax.

Processing tissues to wax with a single reagent

Although there are some reagents that are miscible with water and wax they are not popular in histology. For example, dioxane (diethylene dioxide) can be used as a single bath and will mix completely with water and paraffin wax. The tissue can be simply taken from the fixative (which is usually a water-based solution) and placed in dioxane. The dioxane will then replace the water, though a couple of changes of solution may be needed to completely remove all the water from the tissue. Once all the water has been removed the tissue can then be transferred into molten wax which can then replace the dioxane. Again, more than one bath of reagent is needed to completely remove all the dioxane. Unfortunately dioxane has problems: in particular it is quite toxic, it is relatively expensive and the final results are poorer than using other methods. For these reasons it has never become a common or popular method despite its relative simplicity.

Replacement of tissue water with wax using two intermediate steps

Instead of using just a single reagent, double-stage processing is usually used. The first stage removes water (dehydration) and the second stage replaces the dehydrating agent with a reagent which is miscible with wax (termed clearing). The tissues are then impregnated with wax, placed in a mould and the wax solidified. Sections can be cut from the wax block and then stained. Calcified tissues such as bone are extremely brittle in their natural state but can be decalcified to leave only the soft tissue matrix of bone (osteoid) which can then be processed normally. Figure 3.1 shows how the steps are arranged. Each of these steps will be considered in more detail but it is important to grasp the general scheme of processing tissues.

Reagents for tissue dehydration

In choosing any reagent there are various properties that need to be considered. These are cost, safety, speed of action and its effect on tissues. The speed of action is controlled by the viscosity of the solvent. Dehydration, like most of processing, is really a diffusion process with the solvent diffusing into the tissue and the water diffusing out. The rate of diffusion into a relatively compact structure such as tissue is more dependent on the viscosity of the liquid than on simple molecular weight. Water has a viscosity of 1 cP and higher numbers mean more viscous (thicker) fluids which will penetrate more slowly.

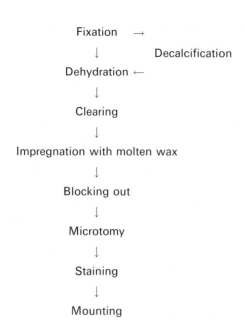

Fixation → Decalcification
↓
Dehydration ←
↓
Clearing
↓
Impregnation with molten wax
↓
Blocking out
↓
Microtomy
↓
Staining
↓
Mounting

Figure 3.1 *Flow of specimen in processing. The fixed specimen is either transferred to dehydrating agents directly or, if there is any mineralized bone present, it is decalcified first before being dehydrated. The dehydration, clearing and impregnation with wax are often done by a machine and can be considered as a single stage called processing*

Safety considerations include both toxicity and flammability. Most of these solvents will burn but their flash points and fire risks vary. The properties of some dehydrating agents are listed in Table 3.1.

As with many steps in histological processing, the more rapid the removal of water the harsher the effect on the tissues. This applies equally to the inherent speed of the reagent and to the graded series of strengths of the reagent. Very gradual removal with a slow reagent may damage the tissues less than rapid removal with a harsher reagent. It is always a trade-off between speed and quality.

Table 3.1 *Properties of dehydrating agents*

Reagent	Cost (£ per litre) at 1997 prices)	Viscosity	Toxicity	Fire hazard	
Ethanol (IMS, 74OP)	£3.40	1.2	?	+	Commonest reagent
Methanol	£2.40	0.6	++	+	Faster and harsher
Propanol	£5.00	2.5	+	+	Slower
Acetone	£3	0.4	++	++	Faster and harsh
Cellosolve (2-ethoxy-ethanol)	£9		+	+	Slower and gentler but destroys some elements
1-Epoxy-propane (propylene oxide)	£8		++ Carcinogen	+++	Used in EM; inhibits some stains
2,2-Dimethoxy-propane	£56		+	++	Reacts with water to form methanol/acetone

Alcohol is unusual amongst laboratory chemicals in also being a foodstuff. It is included in the diets of many people. It is toxic in large quantities but it has been suggested that it may actually prolong life if taken in small quantities by reducing the risk of cardiovascular disease. It seems unlikely that this protective effect will occur with occupational exposure.

Alcohol is also not seriously damaging to the skin and is the basis of many perfumes and aftershave lotions. The alcohol will slightly dry the skin by removing some of the natural oils and is also extremely painful if applied to cuts.

Ethanol is cheap to produce but has the problem that the Customs and Excise people take a great deal of interest, and duty, in anything alcoholic. Although laboratories can get the alcohol with reduced duty they must keep accurate records to show that the alcohol is not being used illicitly. This explains the use of IMS instead of pure and potentially drinkable ethanol. Sometimes alcohol is referred to as 74OP spirit. This again is due to the Customs and Excise who used to test alcoholic spirits to 'prove' them. 100° proof spirit was originally the lowest strength of alcohol which, if it was poured on gunpowder, would allow it to ignite. This was the original 'proof' of the spirits strength. Anything stronger could be diluted and still pass the test, so it was overproof (OP) spirit. Pure alcohol is equivalent to 174° proof hence 74OP.

Although alcohol is the commonest dehydrating reagent it is by no means the only material which can be used. Table 3.1 shows some of the alternatives and their properties.

Ethanol

Ethanol (see Box) has long been used for removing water and is so ubiquitous in laboratories that if a method uses the term alcohol it will mean ethanol rather than any other alcohol. It is quite a gentle reagent compared to many other agents that can be used. Its almost universal use is probably due to its low cost and low toxicity with little tissue damage. Ethanol will remove some materials from the tissue but usually these same materials are removed by all dehydrating and clearing agents so it is not a problem unique to ethanol. Ethanol can be regarded as almost non-toxic in use since the amounts liable to be ingested or inhaled, provided reasonable care is taken, are well below the levels known to cause damage.

In the process of dehydration it is usual to remove the water in a series of steps by using several baths of alcohol of gradually increasing strength ('graded series'). If the specimen is placed directly into concentrated alcohol then the tissue shrinks more and may become excessively hard. The actual concentrations of alcohol used in the graded series vary from laboratory to laboratory. Some processing schedules start with quite weak mixtures (30% alcohol) and increase the strength very slowly whilst others begin at 70% and move quickly to even higher concentrations. Most laboratories get good results which suggests that any differences are small. It is usual to treat delicate tissues such as embryos with a more gradual removal since they are more easily damaged. Very tough tissues, however, may also benefit from a slower, gentler processing to prevent them becoming even tougher. Tough tissues can also be softened by adding other reagents to the dehydrating agents. The addition of phenol can have a beneficial effect on very tough materials.

Methanol

Methanol is important not only as a dehydrating agent in its own right but also because it is added to ethanol to give industrial methylated spirit (IMS) which is not drinkable (see Box) and so has a lower cost and is less strictly controlled than pure ethanol. Methanol is somewhat harsher than ethanol but is also faster and is sometimes used for rapid processing.

Higher alcohols such as propanol and butanol can be used as dehydrating agents but have no great advantages and are only occasionally used for specialized techniques where ethanol and methanol are unsuitable.

Acetone

Acetone like methanol is occasionally used alone since it will dehydrate more quickly than other reagents but it does shrink and harden the tissue much more than ethanol. Acetone is also used more in electron microscopy (EM) than simple ethanol as it is more easily miscible with the plastic resins used in EM. In EM the hardening is less of a problem as the resin gives stronger support than wax and shrinkage is usually less as the fixatives used in EM harden the tissues more than the usual fixatives for wax processing. Acetone will dissolve more materials from the tissues than ethanol and is more of a danger as it has a low flash point and is more toxic than ethanol.

Propylene oxide

The use of this compound is almost entirely restricted to EM and even there some workers prefer to avoid it as it has a very high toxicity compared to other dehydrating agents. The miscibility of propylene oxide with resins is its only real advantage over other agents.

Cellosolve

Cellosolve has the reputation of being gentler than other reagents; tissues may be left in cellosolve for long periods without becoming excessively hard, and it has been recommended for embryos. Generally it is not popular because of its cost. It does easily absorb water from the air so careful storage is essential.

2,2-Dimethoxy-propane

The final dehydrating agent on the list is an oddity as it acts differently. 2,2-Dimethoxy-propane dehydrates the tissues not by simply washing the water out of the tissues and replacing it by diffusion of the dehydrating agent into the tissue spaces, but actually reacting endothermically to produce acetone and methanol. I have never used it and I don't know of anyone who has used it, and this may have something to do with the very high cost.

Ensuring complete dehydration

Complete dehydration is essential since the clearing reagents and waxes are usually intolerant of even small amounts of water. To ensure complete removal of all the water it is important to have at least two baths of 100% alcohol (quite often three or even more are used). The first 100% alcohol bath rapidly becomes contaminated with small amounts of water carried over from the previous lower concentration (e.g. 95% alcohol) bath. The second bath effectively

Clearing agents, as well as being dangerous to use, are also dangerous to dispose of. Many are flammable and can be burnt but this requires very high temperatures and is not practicable for most laboratories. Passing the waste on to a specialist disposal firm is often the best alternative but does carry a high cost. This cost of disposal should be added to the purchase cost when considering which agent to use.

An alternative for large laboratories is recycling of the waste material. Specialist closed stills are available that will redistil solvents, including alcohol and most clearing agents. The capital costs can be high as they need a special room and careful monitoring to ensure safety. Providing the throughput is high enough they can repay the costs in a couple of years. Recycling can be dangerous if picric acid is used since it is explosive.

Even very small amounts of clearing agents should not be allowed to get into the normal waste-disposal system as they will not be effectively rinsed away and diluted. They are not miscible with water and will remain in the traps of sinks. Xylene tends to float, so a layer of xylene will remain floating on the trap and the fumes will be released. The constant exposure to small amounts of solvents will degrade rubber and plastic components of the waste system and produce leaks.

removes all the water. It is still essential to replace the reagents regularly since there will always be a gradual transfer of water from one bath to the next. Some laboratories use anhydrous copper sulphate to test for water in the alcohols. When the alcohol is dry the copper sulphate remains white but when water gets into the alcohol it will turn blue and the reagent needs to be changed. To save on reagent costs it is common to simply move these reagents one step lower down when they become slightly contaminated, so only the final 100% alcohol is replaced by fresh reagent. The old final bath becomes the next to final bath and so on.

Safety is very important with dehydrating agents since they are used in such large quantities. Alcohol has a relatively low toxicity whilst propylene oxide is very toxic. For this reason many people are turning away from propylene oxide even in EM. Fire risks are also important since most laboratories now use electrically driven machines and these may produce sparks. I know of at least two laboratories that caught fire and burnt down from fires starting in the processing rooms.

Clearing

Clearing is the next step and involves the removal of the dehydrating agent, usually alcohol, and its replacement with a solvent miscible with wax. It was originally named thus because many of the reagents had a similar refractive index (RI) to tissues and so cleared them optically (as xylene does). Optical clearing means that the tissues become transparent once they are completely permeated by the reagent. Even though most modern reagents do not clear optically they are still usually referred to as clearing agents (perhaps because they 'clear' the alcohol out of the tissues). Other names have been suggested (e.g. antemedia or de-alcoholizing reagents) but the term clearing is still the most common. For hand-processing of tissues there is still an advantage in optical clearing since it allows the person processing the tissue to see how clearing is progressing, and when the tissue is completely transparent then it is certain that clearing is complete.

Clearing agents

Many organic solvents can act as clearing agents and again there are many agents that have been used and they all have their own advantages and problems (see Table 3.2). Several properties are crucial in evaluating the usefulness of reagents:

- **Speed.** Two factors are included: firstly the speed of removal of alcohol from the tissues and secondly the speed of evaporation of the clearing agent from the wax bath. The speed of removal from wax is related to the boiling point of the clearing agent.

Table 3.2 *Properties of clearing agents*

Clearing agent	Cost per litre	Boiling point (°C)	Refractive index	Toxicity	Flammability
Toluene	£3.40	110.6	1.5	++	++
Xylene	£3.80	138	1.5	+++	++
Chloroform	£4.70	61.5	1.45	++	−
Cedarwood oil	£45	variable	1.5	0	weakly
Petrol hydrocarbons	£4.50	157		+	++
1,1,1-Trichloroethane	£11.30	75	1.43	+	−

- **Harshness of action** and how much **shrinkage or hardening** they cause.
- **Flammability.**
- **Toxicity.**
- **Cost.**

Whereas alcohol is universally used as a routine dehydrating agent there is still variation in which clearing agent is used routinely in different laboratories. Clearing agents are generally much more toxic than alcohol and being volatile they need to be treated with caution. It is generally toxicity that forces the change from one solvent to another rather than poor section quality. For many years benzene was the clearing agent used by many laboratories but the finding that it increases the risk of leukaemia in people exposed to the vapour makes it less popular for use and almost all laboratories stopped using it many years ago.

Toluene

Toluene (methyl benzene) was used as a replacement for benzene but again suffers from toxicity. It is similar in many respects to xylene but not as popular.

Xylene

Many people still use xylene which has a lower toxicity than benzene but is still quite toxic. Xylene is less used in preparing blocks as its harsh action leaves tissues more brittle and harder than many other clearing agents, but it is still very popular for clearing sections after staining where the hardness and brittleness are less of a disadvantage.

Chlorinated solvents

Chlorinated solvents have also been used. Carbon tetrachloride (tetrachloromethane) was quite popular at one time as it is almost non-flammable (it was used in fire extinguishers) but it has severe hepatotoxicity problems. Chloroform (trichloromethane) has a similar toxicity but is still used by some laboratories. 1,1,1-Trichloroethane (used as a dry-cleaning fluid) has a lower toxicity and is often sold as a commercial solution combined with inhibitors which are said to reduce its toxicity. It is, however, now being restricted as it adversely affects the ozone layer, so its use will decline.

Chlorinated hydrocarbons are usually denser and heavier than other clearing agents. This has two consequences. First, and most obviously, they are heavier to lift and secondly many tissues will float in them. This is worth remembering if a cassette holding tissues falls open in the processor, since you need to look in the top of the reagent not at the bottom as you might expect.

Petrol hydrocarbons/aliphatic hydrocarbons

These are now being promoted as a safer alternative to xylene. They seem to be suitable for tissue processing but have problems as clearing agents before coverslipping since they are less miscible with common mounting media.

Cedarwood oil

Although cedarwood oil is no longer popular as a clearing agent it is still widely used as an immersion oil in microscopy. There are various grades of cedarwood oil and the type used for immersion is not the same grade as used for clearing. The immersion oil is thickened compared to the type used for clearing.

This is a slow-acting clearing agent which has very little hardening effect on tissues. It is a very traditional clearing agent and was highly rated in the past but is hardly used at all now because of its cost and slowness. It has a distinctive odour and it never seems to disappear completely from the wax, so the blocks have a faint but pleasant odour. Although it will burn it does not readily catch fire and is not a real fire risk.

Many other reagents have been tried as clearing agents including simple petrol (inflammable but cheap), cooking oil (cheap and hopefully non-toxic), and essential oils such as lavender oil or sandalwood oil (very expensive but the laboratory smells lovely).

Which agent to use

No one material has so far emerged as a clear winner. Each laboratory has different priorities. For some laboratories price is more important than getting the very best quality whereas others want perfection regardless of cost. Some laboratories use such small amounts of clearing agent that toxicity and flammability can be controlled and so it is less of a worry. Other laboratories use solvents on an industrial scale and need to consider safety in a different way.

The dehydrating agent must be completely removed from the tissues, so three or more baths of clearing agent are needed to ensure complete replacement. Reagents need to be regularly changed as already mentioned for the alcohols; again the final bath can be reused as an earlier bath to save replacing all the reagents at once.

Impregnation with molten wax

After clearing is complete the tissues are passed through two to four baths of fresh molten wax. The wax is held at no more than 2–3°C above its melting point rather than at much higher temperatures since heat is very damaging to tissues.

Different waxes have different melting points. Usually a wax with a melting point in the range 55–60°C is used. As a general rule the higher the melting point of the wax the harder the wax is at room temperature. Ideally the hardness of the wax and the hardness of the tissue should be the same, so that the texture of the wax and the block are even and when a section is cut the knife moves smoothly through the block and does not 'jump' on encountering a different texture. In most laboratories a compromise is used with one hardness being used for most specimens. The slight differences in texture between one tissue and the next are usually small enough to be ignored. There may, however, be differences between laboratories because the types of specimens may be quite different. A laboratory dealing mainly with bone will have a different requirement to one which is dealing mainly with brain.

There are also specialist waxes which have additives (such as plasticizers) or microcrystalline waxes to aid in the cutting. These are available ready-prepared and are usually known by their commercial names.

Removal of clearing agents

The clearing agent needs to be completely removed from the final wax bath. If some persists in the block it will later evaporate from the surface of the block. The block may initially cut quite well but after a few days or weeks the tissue will shrink, leaving the surface concave and below the surface of the wax. Although this can be prevented by covering the cut surface of a block with a layer of wax it is better to properly process the block.

The clearing agent is not just washed out of the tissue by the wax bath it is also removed by evaporation. The wax bath is often at a high enough temperature to cause significant amounts of the clearing agent to 'boil off'. This evaporation is often the most sensitive way to tell when the final wax bath needs changing. If the final wax smells of clearing agent then it needs changing.

Evaporation of the clearing agent and removal of air bubbles can be helped by using reduced pressure in the final wax bath(s); this is called 'vacuum embedding' though a true vacuum is not needed, simply a significantly reduced pressure (about 50–75% of atmospheric pressure will suffice).

Blocking out originally used L-shaped brass blocks (Leuckhart's angles) which could be moved to make a variable sized mould. The wax rapidly cools and solidifies so a fluid-tight seal is not needed.

After cooling the blocks were trimmed with a scalpel or small knife and then attached to a fibre or wood block by melting the lower surface and pressing on to the surface. It was easy to get the labels mixed up with so many separate steps.

Then came disposable moulds and the integrated cassette and mould system which is now common. The blocks are now directly mounted on the cassette they were processed in and the cassette fits a special holder in the microtome. There is less scope for a mix-up, the blocks are more rapidly dealt with and throughput is greater.

Blocking-out used to be done with ordinary forceps heated in a Bunsen flame, on a standard bench with wax melted in a beaker in the wax oven which had to be poured manually into the mould. Wax at 60°C is just painful to hold so blocking out was a real pain!

Now there are integrated work-stations with hot wax in a container with a tap, cooled and warmed areas for orienting and cooling the blocks and electrically heated forceps. This is much more efficient.

Blocking-out of tissues

Once all the clearing agent has been removed the tissue is blocked-out in a mould containing fresh wax. It is oriented so that the correct surface will be cut in microtomy and the block is then cooled quickly. Rapid cooling prevents larger wax crystals forming and makes the block more homogeneous and improves the cutting qualities of the block.

Once the tissue is embedded in wax it remains stable, so the next stages can be performed slowly, allowing careful preparation of fine sections. The block can also be stored for many years without deterioration. For unusual or important specimens the blocks can be stored indefinitely and often prove a useful source of retrospective material for research.

Hand versus automatic processing

It is possible to process tissues manually or using an automated schedule on an automatic tissue processor.

Hand processing

Tissues can be processed by hand using a series of containers with the various reagents in sequence. This requires somebody to transfer the tissues. It is tedious but very flexible (each tissue is treated differently). It is generally slower since there is not constant agitation of the reagent. Agitation constantly mixes the reagent which means that there is never a layer of spent reagent next to the block. If left without agitation the reagent diffusing out of the specimen will form a static stagnant layer around the tissue and slow down the processing.

Hand processing is cheap to implement and is still used by laboratories with a very small throughput of blocks. Even large laboratories may occasionally use hand processing for unusual specimens where setting up an automatic processor for a single specimen would be impractical.

Automated processing

Automatic processing uses a machine to carry out all the changes and includes some method of programming so that the time in each reagent can be controlled. Typically about 12 changes of reagent are accommodated by a single machine and times in the baths can be varied from a few minutes up to several hours. The machines are intended to run unsupervised so that processing can be done overnight. The start can also be delayed so that the machine can run over a weekend without the specimens being left too long in the final reagent.

The machines usually have facilities for thermostatically controlled wax baths and many can apply a partial vacuum to one or more steps. This allows the machine to do the complete processing schedule, taking the specimens from fixative right through to wax impregnation. Schedules can be changed quickly and easily and may be computer/microprocessor controlled. This makes processing very easy. Specimens are put on to the machine and can then be left unattended. Many laboratories have the schedules arranged so that a specimen put on to the machine in an afternoon will complete the processing schedule the following morning and be ready for blocking-out into moulds when staff arrive. Paraffin processing often looks complex when written down but is extremely easy with a machine to do the tedious work.

Many specimens (up to hundreds in large machines) are processed simultaneously. Each specimen is placed in a labelled cassette to keep it separate from all the others and a batch of cassettes is put on to the machine. The actual structure and mechanism of the machines differ. In some the reagents are in large beakers and the specimens are held in a basket which is then moved from one beaker to the next. In other machines there is only one bath into which the specimens are placed and the reagents are then pumped into and out of the chamber. This allows a sealed system and a vacuum can be applied to the bath. Both types have similar applications and it is only cost and the number of specimens that are different.

Automatic processing is generally faster, more reliable, more convenient and can be done overnight with no problems. It is less flexible since all the specimens in one batch get the same times regardless of size, fixation, consistency etc. Regular agitation is usual so the results are faster and more consistent. This is used for laboratories with larger numbers of blocks which are fairly similar in size and texture. If the laboratory is large enough then it may be able to justify several automatic processors set up with a variety of schedules so that individual blocks can get more specialized treatment.

Decalcification

Tissues such as bone and teeth are strengthened and hardened by the addition of a mineral which consists of a mixture of calcium and phosphate and hydroxide with smaller amounts of magnesium, potassium, chlorides and carbonates. This mineral is hydroxyapatite. In bone about 70% of the tissue is mineral, in dentine about 97% is mineral and tooth enamel is over 99% mineral. The hydroxyapatite is quite hard and makes routine sectioning difficult. The tissue can be softened by removing the mineral, and this process is usually called decalcification though it also removes materials other than just calcium.

The use of flammable liquids such as alcohols and hydrocarbons in processing make it quite a fire risk. This is especially true once the system becomes automated. Automatic processors are electric and have electrically heated wax baths. A spark from an electric motor or thermostat can easily result in a major fire. To prevent this most modern machines are completely enclosed and the vapours are prevented from escaping by always using a partial vacuum so that the air flow is into the chamber. The reagents are pumped into and out of this evacuated chamber and stored in sealed containers when not in use. Older machines which used relatively open baths of reagents were always a fire risk. Some laboratories were destroyed by fire which also meant the loss of irreplaceable diagnostic tissue samples.

The very high mineral content of enamel makes it almost impossible to decalcify teeth and still retain the enamel layer. The enamel has almost no organic content to hold it together so once the mineral disappears the enamel layer becomes very fragile and falls apart. Enamel and dentine can also be decalcified *in situ* in the mouth by the acids produced by bacteria. Teeth are also attacked by highly acidic drinks such as lemon juice or cola. Cola drinks contain phosphoric acid and may have a pH of around pH 4. This is quite low enough to be used as a decalcifying solution.

Decalcification with acid solutions

The hydroxyapatite is soluble at low pH and can be removed by treating the tissues with acid:

$$Ca_{10}(PO_4)_6(OH)_2 = 10\,Ca^{2+} + 6\,PO_4^{3-} + 2\,OH^-$$

The mineral is usually in equilibrium with the body fluids but if the pH is lowered then the excess hydrogen ions combine with the hydroxyl ions to give water. This removal of the hydroxyl ions drives the reaction to the right, giving a net result of:

$$Ca_{10}(PO_4)_6(OH)_2 + 20\,H^+ = 10\,Ca^{2+} + 6\,H_3PO_4 + 2\,H_2O$$

The calcium ions will form salts with whatever acid is being used (e.g. calcium chloride with hydrochloric acid).

Acid solutions damage soft tissues

Mineral acids such as hydrochloric acid and nitric acid are generally faster than organic acids but cause more **maceration** of the tissues. Maceration involves swelling of tissues, loss of staining ability and generally poorer morphology. The maceration is caused simply by the hydrogen ions causing hydrolysis of proteins and nucleic acids and is worse if the tissue is inadequately fixed. Although thorough fixation minimizes the effects of the maceration it cannot totally prevent some deterioration. Maceration is also increased by leaving tissues in acid for longer than necessary or using higher temperatures to speed up decalcification. Decalcification is always a compromise between speed and quality of morphology.

Acid decalcifying solutions

Different acid decalcifying solutions give a choice between quality and speed. Acids which are used in practice include:

- **Nitric acid** (e.g. Perenyi's fluid). This is very fast-acting but causes severe maceration if used for more than a few hours. It is only suitable for very urgent cases. Old stocks of nitric acid often turn a yellowish colour and this exaggerates the disruption and also stains the tissue. The addition of urea is sometimes recommended to help prevent the disruption and discoloration.

- **Hydrochloric acid** has been used and is often a part of commercial or proprietary decalcifying solutions. Although it works well it does cause maceration though not as badly as nitric acid. It should not be mixed with formaldehyde as it can produce a carcinogen.

- **Formic acid** is probably the most common decalcifying acid and is used at a concentration of between 5 and 30%. It is significantly slower than the mineral acids but causes less damage.

- **Acetic acid and peracetic acid** can also be used but are even slower than formic acid but do not adversely affect nuclear staining.

Some acids are unsuitable as decalcifying agents. Sulphuric acid for example forms insoluble calcium sulphate which is then extremely difficult to remove.

Chelating agents as non-acidic decalcifying solutions

An alternative to using acids is to use a chelating agent. These decalcify by continuously removing the small amount of free ionic calcium which is always present around the bone mineral. This removal acts in the same way as the removal of OH ions drives the equilibrium to the right in the equation on p. 30.

It is, however, much slower in action. The main chelating agent used is EDTA (ethylenediaminetetraacetic acid). Since this reaction can occur at neutral pH there is no damage to fixed tissue and preservation is excellent but decalcification is very slow (it may take months to completely decalcify larger pieces of bone or teeth).

Many attempts have been made to speed up decalcification

Acceleration of decalcification is possible but some methods also accelerate maceration. The most effective action is regular replacement of decalcifying solution. This replenishes the acidity and speeds up decalcification. Simple agitation to prevent the layer of fluid around the specimen becoming saturated with the calcium is also very effective. This does not really require constant agitation, just an occasional shake seems to work well, though any gentle automatic agitation will be beneficial.

Heating the solution certainly speeds up the reaction but also speeds up the maceration reactions so there is no real benefit in using heat. The use of electrical currents (electrolysis) and ultrasonic treatment seem to speed up the reaction but this seems to be mainly due to their heating effects rather than any more subtle effect. If the solutions are kept cool then there is no real increase in speed.

By using an organic acid in a buffered state it is possible to keep the hydrogen ion concentration more uniform. As the hydroxide ions neutralize the hydrogen ions in an unbuffered solution the rate of decalcification falls as the pH rises. In a buffer the hydrogen ions are replaced at the same rate as they are removed so decalcification is more evenly paced.

The inclusion of an ion-exchange resin in the solution has been used to try and give the same replenishing effect. They seem to be rather more tedious to use than simply buffering the solution since the resin needs to be regenerated after use. Ion-exchange resins can

Undecalcified sections are needed when the actual process of bone mineralization is being investigated. This occurs in bone disease such as osteoporosis. There is no theoretical difference between undecalcified bone sections and soft-tissue sectioning but the practical problems and difficulties are much greater with the rigid and brittle mineralized tissues. They can also be prepared by the totally different method of ground sections. In this technique, rather than removing a section from a block by microtomy the thin section is prepared by removing all the unwanted block by grinding it away. One side of the specimen is ground flat and then attached to a slide. The exposed side of the block is then ground away until the required thinness is achieved. This is quite wasteful of tissue as only one section is prepared from each block. Machines to automatically grind sections are available as this is the standard way of making geological slides from rock samples. In fact geologists consider bone to be very soft rather than hard. I suppose it is if you compare it to granite.

only be used with organic acids and they prevent the use of the chemical end-point test.

Buffering is advantageous and one of the best decalcifying agents is a mixture of formic acid and trisodium citrate. The citrate acts as a buffer salt and also as a chelating agent. The pH is quite moderate and causes minimal maceration but it is still quite a slow decalcifying solution.

Decalcification in fixatives

Acids must of course be avoided if the bone is to be examined as undecalcified specimens. Sources of acid in processing include acetic and peracetic acids, picric acid and unbuffered formaldehyde solutions (these may contain formic acid). Fixatives containing acetic acid and picric acid will decalcify very small fragments of bone during fixation. This can be useful for bone marrow specimens where there may be a few tiny fragments of bone present but it is not worthwhile doing a full decalcification. Fixation in a fixative containing acetic acid softens the tiny fragments, allowing the tissue to be cut but without delaying the specimen.

Accurate determination of the end-point of decalcification

The 'end-point' of decalcification is the moment when the last calcium deposit is removed leaving only the soft tissues. The end-point needs to be accurately determined so that the specimen is removed from the destructive acid bath as soon as possible in order to minimize the maceration caused by excessive exposure to acids. The end-point can be determined by several methods.

X-rays

This is probably the most accurate method but is inconvenient for most laboratories. Tissues are placed on top of an X-ray film in a light-tight cassette and then exposed to sufficient X-rays to make the film very dark but not quite completely black. Any calcium deposits show as white areas on the developed X-ray film while soft tissues appear as a faint grey background. It can be expensive as it requires X-ray films. It can be used to show how decalcification is proceeding, as well as indicating when it is complete.

Chemical testing

Chemical testing of the fluid can be carried out to see if calcium is present. A sample of the decalcifying fluid is taken and neutralized with hydroxide solution. Adding ammonium oxalate to this neutralized solution will show if calcium is present by producing a precipitate which appears slightly hazy if viewed against a dark background. If calcium is detected then it means that decalcification is still proceeding and the decalcifying fluid should be changed and retested a few hours later. Once there is no faint precipitate it can be taken that decalcification is complete.

Manual testing

This includes testing by bending or poking with a needle (NOT recommended). Although it is possible to detect calcified tissue by its rigidity this method can cause damage to the tissue, especially if it is repeated many times.

Following decalcification the block should be washed free of acid in either a sodium sulphate solution or alcohol (simply washing in water causes further swelling) and then the tissue can be processed as for soft tissue.

A slightly better method of using poking is to set up a decalcification using a test piece of bone the same size as the specimen and decalcify it in parallel with the specimen. This piece of bone can be bent, needled and even cut to see if it is decalcified. When the test sample is decalcified the other piece is assumed to be completed as well. It is not really all that accurate as the density of the bones will not be identical but it is useful as a guide.

Microtomy

The wax blocks can be cut using a microtome. This is a finely engineered machine capable of slicing sections regularly at 5 μm or less. Microtomes come in many types from small hand-held ones to extremely large ones that can fill a small room. They all have certain characteristics in common:

- A mechanism for holding the block firmly. The block is usually attached to a holder or chuck and this is clamped in a jaw mechanism.
- A knife holder.
- A mechanism to move the knife across the surface of the block to cut a section.
- A feed mechanism to advance the block so that a subsequent section can be cut at the required thickness.

The engineering ingenuity which has gone into achieving these characteristics is quite remarkable and most microtomists have their own favourite types of microtome.

Some microtomes are better for particular purposes. The things that make one microtome better, or at least better for one purpose, are controlled mainly by the specimen and what is required from it. Considerations include:

- **How big is the block?** The bigger the block the larger the microtome needed, but large microtomes can be very inconvenient for small specimens.
- **How hard is the block?** Very hard blocks of bone or tooth need a specialized microtome but such machines are usually somewhat tedious to use for soft specimens.
- **Are serial sections needed?** Serial sections are where several adjacent sections are cut in order to follow structures, e.g.

nerves, through the tissue or where exactly adjacent sections are used to apply more than one staining technique to the one specimen. A microtome which can give ribbons is best for such work.

● Cost.

Microtome types

Hand microtomes

These are very simple with a small, flat circular table around a central hollow pillar. The specimen is placed in the centre of the pillar and can be gradually inched up above the table. (It should be 'micrometred' up but that doesn't sound right in English.) By slicing across, using the table as a guide plate, thin sections can be cut. These are not suitable for serious histology and are mainly used for relatively thick sections of botanical specimens.

Rocking microtomes

These are quite small microtomes with two rocking arms. One arm gives the cutting action whilst the other acts as a feed mechanism. These small microtomes were once very common but have largely disappeared from laboratory use but are still used as 'student microtomes' since they are cheap and robust. They are limited to cutting small blocks and soft tissue since the actual cutting action is done by a spring. They were also very popular in cryostats (see Chapter 5) since they have no sliding parts (the only movement is a rocking movement) and so they had no problems with lubrication at the low temperatures in a cryostat (even thin oils become very sticky at $-20°C$).

Rotary microtomes

These are more robust microtomes with a rotating handle. They are very popular in laboratories and come in a variety of sizes. They can produce nice ribbons of sections, are quite reliable if well maintained but can be prone to wear if badly maintained and then they can be quite erratic in use. Once you get familiar with them they can be very easy and quick to use. Not quite as good for very large or very hard blocks as a sliding microtome.

Sliding microtomes

These are usually much heavier and larger machines than the other types. The cutting action is by sliding a heavy 'sledge' under a knife. These can cut very large and very hard blocks but are heavier to use as a consequence. They are quite popular and in some laboratories they are used to cut all specimens, even small soft ones.

Microtome knives

The knife used in a microtome is equally important and it must be very sharp and the edge must be free from blemishes. Knives can be solid and need sharpening or they can be disposable. Solid knives can be sharpened by hand, though this is no longer common, or sharpened by machines.

There is no great difficulty in understanding how knives are sharpened as it is fairly straightforward and logical. Sharpening involves removing metal from the edge of the knife to create a new sharp cutting edge. Large nicks are removed using a coarse abrasive (silicon carbide, also known as carborundum, or diamond powders) and then using finer abrasives to remove the scratches left by the coarse abrasives. Hand grinding usually uses hones or sharpening stones of different grades.

Sharpening machines can use powders (suspended in water or oil) and a hard glass or metal plate. These types of machine suffer from the fact that as the plate wears away the metal of the knife to sharpen it, so the knife also wears away the material of the plate and thus causes it to lose its original flat surface. The knives gradually become curved instead of having a straight edge.

The most popular sharpening machines now use a soft metal plate into which a diamond paste is rubbed. The plate becomes studded with very fine diamond particles and the knife is now sharpened on a thin layer of diamond which is regularly renewed and the plate itself does not wear away. This does need several plates, however, since each plate represents one grade of abrasive and you cannot mix coarse and fine abrasives on the same plate.

While sharpening is occurring the knife is wearing away. Since the knife is held at a constant angle this means that the knife develops a facet which is the actual cutting edge. The facet grows larger with constant sharpening, so the knife becomes more difficult to sharpen and sections become more difficult to cut. Eventually the knife becomes unusable for fine sectioning and is either relegated to 'trimming' or is reground to give a new small facet but at a different angle.

Very acute angles of facet are 'sharper' but lose their sharpness more quickly. Thin edges are less rigid and when used with hard blocks they may produce 'chattering'. Chatters are where the section thickness varies across the block as the knife edge moves slightly. The final section shows thick and thin stripes. Less acute facets last longer and are more rigid but cannot cut such fine sections.

Disposable knives are gradually taking over from 'solid' knives in routine histology. They involve less capital cost (for example no knife sharpening equipment is needed) and a fresh knife is always available. One of the horrors of the microtomist is when all his knives are damaged at the same time and he is stuck until they are resharpened. Disposable knives possibly cost more in day-to-day

There is nothing that brings out the argumentative side of histologists more than suggesting that the microtome or knife they are using is inferior. The relative benefits and shortcomings of these machines can be discussed at great length.

In reality the only criterion is whether it produces a good section. Most microtomes in the hands of a good microtomist will cut good sections from most blocks. Only with the very hard or very large blocks does the choice of microtome become crucial.

Microtomy has improved greatly over the years and sections are now routinely cut much thinner than a few years ago. The advent of the disposable knife has been a major factor in this improvement.

There are a few unusual types of microtome in some specialist laboratories. The Tetrander and Jung K microtomes were produced for very large and very hard blocks respectively and would not look out of place in a heavy machine shop as they are really substantial instruments.

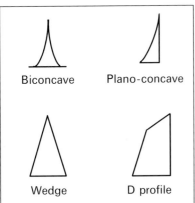

Biconcave   Plano-concave

Wedge   D profile

Solid knives are available in a variety of cross-sectional shapes. The biconcave and plano-concave are good for soft tissues and have a narrow leading edge that can produce an acutely angled and sharp facet. The wedge and D profile knives are more rigid for harder blocks. The wedge shape is usually preferred for frozen sections.

To help cut difficult specimens it is possible to give extra support by covering the surface of the block. The material can be Sellotape or specialized films which polymerize. The Sellotape is pressed firmly on to the face of the block and then as the section is cut the Sellotape and section are lifted off. The sections are then attached to slides using an adhesive but without being floated on to a water bath. The Sellotape is usually removed by using a solvent to dissolve the glue before the section is stained. This method is used for cutting undecalcified bone sections.

A solution of nitrocellulose in alcohol can also be used by painting it on to the block face. This leaves a thin layer of nitrocellulose on the block. This gives less support than the Sellotape but is easier to remove.

running expenses but the ease of use and the fact that it doesn't matter if the knife gets damaged usually outweigh this in a busy laboratory where urgency is paramount.

Very hard blocks need special knives and for very hard specimens the knife can be made of extra hard materials, usually tungsten, and these are not disposable. Also very large specimens are not really catered for by the manufacturers of disposable knives, so non-disposable knives are needed for very large and very hard blocks.

Cutting the section

Cutting is not automatic it needs skill and can be difficult sometimes. It is a practical skill and is best learnt by actually doing it. The things which usually go wrong are:

- **Poor impregnation.** This means the tissue is inadequately supported and will crumble or fold instead of cutting nicely. Poor support can also result from using wax of the wrong temperature (too soft usually) or if the room is too hot, causing the wax to soften. Cooling the block with a block of ice may help.
- **Blunt knife.** Obvious really and usually quite easy to spot in practice.
- **Wrong knife angle.** Probably one of the few things that can be quickly tried during cutting, but once the angle is right it doesn't usually need to be changed between blocks.
- **Slackness in the microtome.** This results in alternate thick and thin sections or in chattering depending on how much slackness or unwanted movement there is.

There are many tricks and dodges which are learnt with practice and experience and no amount of 'book learning' will ever replace just sitting at a microtome and cutting.

Sections can be cut at different thicknesses. Thick sections are useful for low power microscopy, for tracing long structures such as nerves as they travel through tissues and for some histochemical techniques. Thin sections are needed for fine intracellular detail and high power microscopy (especially in photomicrography). For routine wax sections 3–6 µm is usual.

Floating and mounting

All the microtomes have a chopping rather than a cutting action and this has a tendency to compress the section in the direction of cutting. This can result in wrinkles or folds in the section. To get rid of the wrinkles the section is floated on to a bath of warm water. This does not melt the wax but softens it sufficiently for the tissues to recover back to their original shape and size. Gentle prodding with a soft brush can also help to flatten the section. For stubborn wrinkles it is sometimes useful to float the section on to a few drops of alcohol on a slide first and then float it on to the warm water. The turbulence produced as the alcohol mixes with the warm water may sometimes gently ease out the wrinkles.

Sections can then be lifted on to a clean slide. The slide is held in the water bath vertically and the section lifted on to it by withdrawing the slide still held vertically. This works much better than trying to slip the slide horizontally under the section and then trap it on the slide. Withdrawing the slide vertically also traps less water and is less likely to trap air bubbles under the section.

If a ribbon of sections has been cut then either individual sections or a short length of the ribbon containing several sections can be cut from the ribbon either before floating out or on the surface of the waterbath and then picked up as for single sections. The slide should then be labelled. Some slides have ground-glass areas which will accept a soft pencil writing on them but plain slides should be labelled by scratching with a diamond-tipped stylus. Ordinary felt-tip pens, paper labels and most forms of ink will not survive the staining and mounting process and the labelling will be lost.

Once picked up on to a slide the sections are well drained and then dried on to the slide to achieve adhesion. This can be done at any temperature from 37°C to temperatures high enough to melt the wax. Lower temperatures give less damage to the tissue. If the wax melts then the tissue may completely disintegrate. However at 37°C it may need many hours to give complete drying. If drying is incomplete the sections will detach during staining. Most laboratories have their own way and time of drying slides, usually it is higher than 37°C but less than the melting point of the wax used in the laboratory. The drying can be done in an oven or on a hotplate, with the oven method being somewhat slower than using the same temperature with a hotplate, but there is less contamination from dust settling on the slide if it is dried vertically in an oven rather than horizontally on a hotplate on an open bench.

If there are problems with sections adhering or if the staining method is particularly harsh and liable to remove the section then some extra adhesion may be required. Adhesion can be improved by coating the slides and special slides coated with silane (3-aminopropyltriethoxysilane) are available which have a surface charge which helps the section cling to the slide. It is possible to coat ordinary slides with 2% silane in acetone and then drain and dry them but the reagent is quite dangerous.

It is also possible to use chemical adhesives in the form of protein, such as egg albumen, serum, gelatine or poly-L-lysine which are used to coat the slides prior to picking up the sections. Although these do help adhesion they may stain with some techniques, giving a disturbing background.

Suggested further reading

Anderson, G. and Gordon, K.C. (1996). Tissue processing, microtomy and paraffin sections, in *Theory and Practice of Histological Techniques* (eds J.O. Bancroft and A. Stevens). Edinburgh: Churchill Livingstone.

Culling, C.F.A. (1975). *Handbook of Histopathological and Histochemical Techniques*. London: Butterworths.

Self-assessment questions

1. Why are tissues commonly embedded in wax for section cutting?
2. Name, in order, the steps needed to prepare a paraffin wax block.
3. What is a 'graded series' of alcohol and what is its purpose? Name three alternatives to alcohol.
4. How did clearing agents get their name?
5. Name four clearing agents and compare their advantages and problems.
6. What is meant by vacuum embedding?
7. How can mineralized bone be softened for sectioning?
8. Outline how undecalcified bone sections can be prepared.
9. A piece of bone marrow is fixed in a mixture of methanol and acetic acid. Sections of the bone fragments show no sign of calcium.
   Does this indicate that the patient had osteomalacia?
10. Outline the uses and advantages of tungsten knives, disposable knives and plano-concave knives in microtomy.

Key Concepts and Facts

Tissue Support

- Human tissues require support to enable them to be sectioned thinly.

- Different embedding media can act as supports.

Paraffin Wax Embedding

- Paraffin wax is the most common embedding medium for light microscopy.

- Processing for paraffin wax involves dehydration, clearing and impregnation in molten wax.

- Tissues are blocked-out in fresh molten wax, oriented in the mould and then cooled to harden the wax.

- Decalcification is needed to soften mineralized tissues before processing.

- Microtomes are used to prepare thin sections and the sections are flattened on a water bath and finally attached to slides.

Chapter 4
Other embedding techniques

Learning objectives

After studying this chapter you should confidently be able to:

Name alternatives to wax embedding.

Briefly describe the use of plastics (resins) in light and electron microscopy.

Compare the use of methacrylate and epoxy resins.

Outline the benefits and problems of water soluble and ester waxes.

Outline the use of celloidin as a principle embedding medium and also in double embedding.

Although paraffin wax embedding is the commonest method of supporting tissues for sectioning, there are a variety of alternative embedding media which can be used. Some of these are of mainly historical interest whilst others are more recent and are now routine. Even the 'historical' methods have a surprising durability with most of them still being used regularly for specialized purposes and many of them are still useful to overcome some modern research problems. They range from the use of very hard plastics and resins used to produce very thin sections through wax-like materials which have some quite different properties to those of paraffin wax, to the soft and pliable celloidin sections.

Plastic or resin embedding

Plastics are very widely used as embedding media in histology. They are the main embedding method used in electron microscopy and have many applications in light microscopy. The terms plastic and resin tend to be used somewhat loosely in histology. To a chemist all resins are not plastics and not all plastics are resins but for most histologists the terms resin embedding and plastic embedding are simply alternatives.

These materials are usually very much harder than waxes and so give much better support to the tissues. This is better for hard materials such as undecalcified bone and allows much thinner sections to be prepared from soft tissues. Sections may be thinner than 100 nm (about one-fiftieth of the thickness of paraffin sections). This thinness is essential for electron microscopy and can be very useful for light microscopy since there is less confusion from overlapping cells and organelles. One slight problem is the loss of contrast in the sections due to their thinness. This means that staining must be more intense and so staining techniques must be changed for plastic sections. The traditional haematoxylin and eosin is often replaced by using toluidine blue to stain the nucleus and a stronger cytoplasmic stain.

Plastics are quite unlike waxes in one major property. Waxes are converted from a solid to a liquid form by melting and will solidify again on cooling. So tissues are impregnated in molten wax at about 60°C and converted to a solid block by simply cooling. The block can be gently remelted and reblocked without damaging the tissue. Plastics, however, are solidified by chemically converting them from a liquid monomer to a solid polymer. This is irreversible so reblocking is difficult or impossible.

The monomers of the plastics are often miscible with one or more dehydrating agents, particularly acetone and propylene oxide, so that clearing agents such as xylene are often not needed. Some monomers are even miscible with water and the tissue can be impregnated with the monomer directly from aqueous solutions without any need to dehydrate. The miscibility of the monomer and the solubility of the polymer are, however, totally different and once converted to a polymer they are often insoluble. So, for example, glycol methacrylate monomer is miscible with water but once polymerized to the solid polymer the plastic is not only no longer soluble in water but is also insoluble in most other common solvents.

Methacrylates

These are related to perspex and were the first plastic materials to be used for tissue embedding. They were introduced into histology during the early 1950s and have been used in various forms ever since. The early methacrylates were the butyl and methyl methacrylates and then later glycol methacrylate was used (2-hydroxyethyl methacrylate), but since the 1980s aromatic polyhydroxy dimethacrylate resins have been available.

$$CH_2 = \overset{\overset{\displaystyle CH_3}{|}}{\underset{\underset{\displaystyle COOR}{|}}{C}}$$

R = CH₃ — Methyl methacrylate
R = (CH₂)₃CH₃ — Butyl methacrylate
R = (CH₂)₂OH — Glycol methacrylate

The tissue requires dehydration but not clearing since the monomers are miscible with alcohol and acetone. The dehydrating

Methacrylates can also be used for museum specimens since they can be produced in quite large blocks and are crystal clear. The specimen is dehydrated and impregnated as usual but with big specimens the impregnation time is extended. Polymerization must be slow. The block is then trimmed and polished. These embedded specimens are good for teaching since they are less easily damaged than the conventional glass jars filled with fluid. They can get scratched or slightly chipped but don't shatter if dropped. The occasional polish to remove scratches is all that is needed.

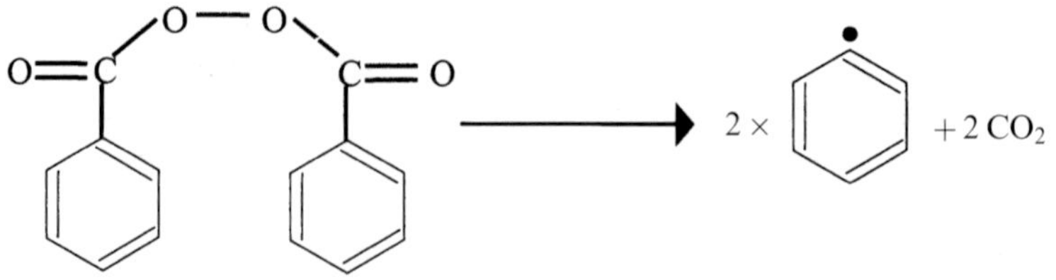

Figure 4.1 *Benzoyl peroxide splitting to give two phenyl radicals*

agent must be completely removed by several changes of monomer before attempting to polymerize the block. Acetone is more of a problem than alcohol for interfering with polymerization and so alcohol is recommended.

Methacrylates polymerize by chain elongation using an active radical. Adding a catalyst such as benzoyl peroxide produces active radicals. This molecule is highly unstable and is explosive but can be obtained as a more stable paste mixed with dibutyl phthalate. When the molecule is heated it can split to provide two stable active radicals (Figure 4.1). The active radical then adds on to a monomer forming a new larger active radical which in turn adds on to a monomer and hence the chain elongates (Figure 4.2). The chain elongation will continue until either there are no free monomers to react or the free radical is inactivated by a free radical scavenger such as oxygen or acetone.

Polymerization of the resin is better if oxygen is removed by bubbling the monomer with nitrogen gas just before use. If the block is not polymerized in a sealed mould then the upper part of the block may not fully polymerize due to the oxygen. Some extra monomer should be used so that this upper soft layer can be removed without harming the embedded tissue.

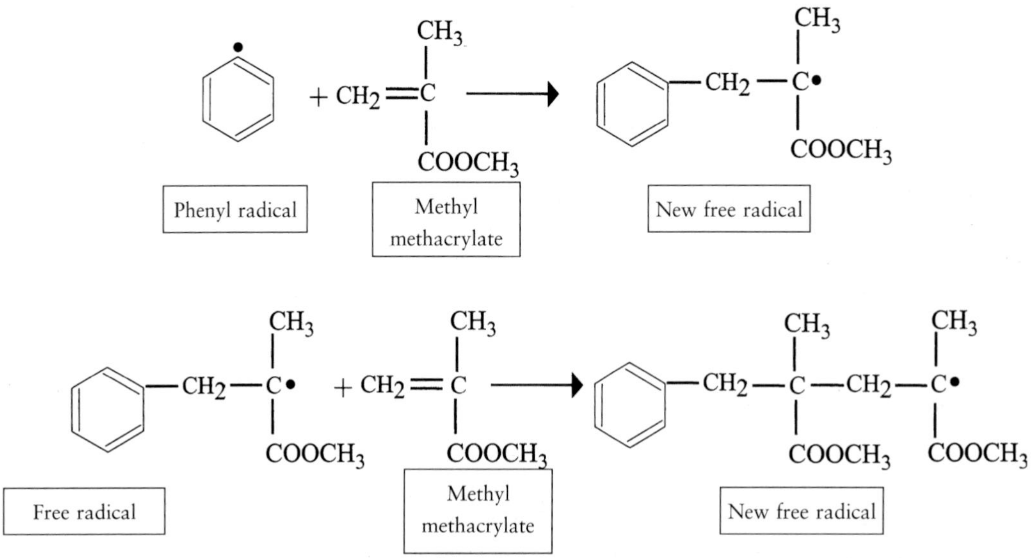

Figure 4.2 *Polymerization of methacrylates*

Rapid high temperature curing will result in more free radicals and the block will suffer as the polymer chains will be shorter. A slower polymerization will give a better result. This is difficult since the reaction needs heat to start it off and once started it is exothermic and will get hotter and hotter, so it is a delicate problem to heat the block enough to start the polymerization and then cool it to remove the heat and slow down the polymerization.

Problems with methyl and butyl methacrylates

Methacrylates have significant problems in use. First they are often sold in an impure form with quinol materials to help stabilize them. These can be removed by extraction of the acrylic monomer with sodium hydroxide. The quinol dissolves in the sodium hydroxide solution which can be discarded. The resin is then washed free of the hydroxide and finally dried with calcium chloride.

The monomer is strongly exothermic and will get very hot during polymerization. To minimize damage to the tissues it is better to do some of the initial polymerization before impregnation. So pre-polymerized monomer is made by starting the polymerization and then cooling the partially polymerized material to 0°C. An alternative is to use some low molecular weight beads dissolved in the monomer. If the heat is not controlled then the heat may get so intense that the monomer may vaporize causing cavities in the block.

Glycol methacrylate (HEMA)

Glycol methacrylate or 2-hydroxy-ethyl methacrylate (HEMA) is a useful addition to the resins since the monomer is hydrophilic and complete removal of water is not essential before impregnating in monomer. The tissue is often only dehydrated to 90% alcohol before being impregnated with the glycol methacrylate monomer. Once completely impregnated with monomer, and this can take two or three changes, it can then be polymerized. Some forms of glycol methacrylate are contaminated with methacrylic acid which can take up stains and this can cause the problem of a heavy background colour. Low acid monomers are preferable. Although the monomer is water soluble the cured resin is insoluble in most reagents and is not easily removed.

Aromatic polyhydroxy methacrylates

Aromatic polyhydroxy methacrylates have been available since the 1980s and have the hydrophilic characteristics of glycol methacrylate but are more stable in the electron microscope. These resins can also be cured by exposure to UV light and can be cured at very low temperatures, allowing some enzyme histochemistry to be done.

Cutting and staining for methacrylates

Acrylic resins can be cut with ordinary steel or disposable knives but better results are usually obtained if they are sectioned using glass knives (see Chapter 16 on Electron microscopy) for thin sections of soft tissue or tungsten knives for sections of hard, undecalcified tissues. Sections can be stained as free-floating sections without removing the plastic or they can be attached to slides using an adhesive and then the methacrylate softened or removed.

Methyl and butyl methacrylate can be dissolved using xylene and so can be stained by a wide variety of techniques similar in fact to paraffin sections. These methacrylates are no longer popular for electron microscopy since the resins disintegrate slowly in the electron beam, but they are still very useful for light microscopy and especially when working with hard tissues such as undecalcified bone and teeth. They are excellent for light microscopy as the resin is easily permeated by aqueous dyes and, in the case of methyl methacrylate, can even be removed by soaking in xylene. (The epoxy resins which are preferred for EM are more difficult to stain and impossible to remove.)

Glycol methacrylate is more difficult to remove and tissues are always stained with the resin still in place. The glycol resin is, however, still hydrophilic and allows penetration of many aqueous dyes so staining is still fairly easy. It is this flexibility of staining with dyes which has meant that acrylic resins have retained their popularity for light microscopy while electron microscopists have largely discarded them.

Epoxy resins

These are commercially produced resins and their exact chemical nature is often a commercial secret. They include Araldite, Epon and Spurr resins. They are generally much more viscous than the acrylic resins but have the advantage of causing very little shrinkage and do not produce damaging heat during polymerization.

The epoxy resins polymerize by a different mechanism involving crosslinking of two different components and are more likely to produce crosslinks between the extending polymer chains. Instead of using just a monomer and a small amount of catalyst they need two major components that interact to form the polymer (Figure 4.3). Other materials can be added as accelerators and plasticizers such as dibutyl phthalate.

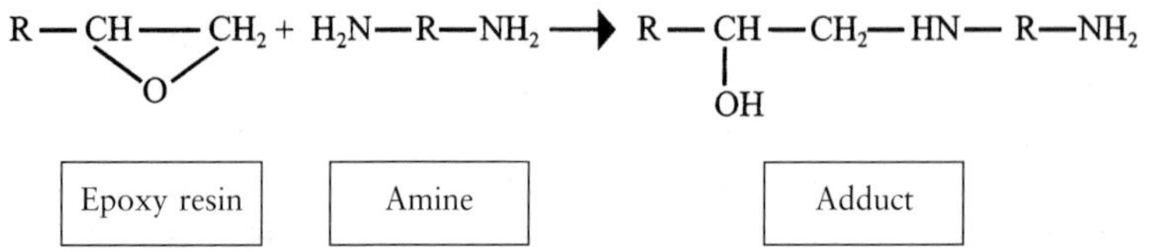

Figure 4.3 *Epoxy resin polymerization. The epoxide group reacts with amines to form adducts. The adduct has amines and an alcohol, both of which can then further react with another epoxide group to give chain elongation and branching*

The curing of these materials alters their characteristics. The higher the temperature the harder the blocks will be and they will also be more brittle. Curing for histology is usually done at 60°C for 12–24 h which gives a tougher but less hard block. At 120°C the block will be cured in 1 h but will be hard and brittle.

Since the components of the resin can bond to amine groups there is the possibility of the plastic bonding directly on to the proteins and nucleic acids in the tissues. The tissue becomes permanently attached to the resin and the degree of crosslinking means that, especially for small blocks, the whole block is essentially just one large extended molecule including the tissues. The result of this is that staining is inhibited and antigens are blocked, so staining with dyes and immunohistochemical techniques are poor. It is almost impossible to remove the resin without destroying the tissue in the process. Some improvement can be obtained by breaking down some of the crosslinks or etching the block with sodium hydroxide in alcohol. Staining is still depressed compared to other embedding techniques.

Epoxy resins can include some very toxic materials and should be treated with care. They are capable of linking on to the tissues in human skin and acting as a hapten group. This slightly alters the nature of the proteins in skin so that the immune system will treat them as foreign proteins and produce an immunity. This results in an allergic hypersensitivity to the resin materials. They should only be used inside a fume cupboard and gloves are needed when the monomers are being handled.

Cutting and staining for epoxy resins

As with the methacrylates it is better to use tungsten or glass knives to cut these materials though it is possible with steel knives. Sections are usually dried on to slides using an adhesive and stained as for paraffin wax sections. As mentioned above, a pretreatment with sodium hydroxide may help the dyes to penetrate a little further but most staining will only occur at the surface rather than throughout the section.

Because they essentially form a single large molecule they are less liable to disintegrate in the electron beam which means they will remain intact for longer and will not contaminate the inside of the electron microscope.

Alternative waxes

These are materials which look and feel like wax but have quite different properties. They have lower melting points than standard paraffin wax but are still strong enough to act as a tissue support. The waxes often need less processing and can accept tissues from dehydrating agents or even water. The result is often fewer artefacts

Water soluble waxes are also used for impregnating many other things to protect and support them. They have the advantage of being easily removed if this becomes necessary and can be applied from either water or from alcoholic solutions. These waxes are being used to protect the 16th century warship the Mary Rose which sank in the Solent in 1545 and was then raised from the sea bed in 1982. Because the timbers were waterlogged and liable to disintegrate if they were allowed to dry, they have been kept moist and then gradually impregnated with polyethylene glycols which will coat and support the wood.

A different medium, hydroxy-propyl cellulose, was found to be the best way to recover the leather bindings of old books and is currently being used in restoring the books in Trinity College Dublin's famous old Long Room Library. They did try using methacrylates to fulfil the same supporting role for the drying and splintering covers but it tended to cause discoloration.

and this can be a big advantage, but they have never really become widely used for routine work because of the cost involved.

Water soluble wax

These are not really waxes at all but polyethylene glycols. They usually have a lower melting point than paraffin wax but are still similar in hardness to the common paraffin waxes used in histology. They are completely soluble in water so tissues can be transferred into them without dehydration. Usually an intermediate bath of 1:1 fixative and polyethylene glycol is used to make the transition more gentle, but it is not essential. The blocks are easy to cut and the tissue shrinks less since there are no dehydration and clearing steps and the impregnation is at a lower temperature. There are fewer artefacts than with the usual paraffin wax (for example lipids can be retained in the section). The reason they are not used very much is that after cutting they are very difficult to handle.

Sections cannot be conveniently floated on to a water bath for the tissue to relax and flatten after the rough action of being 'chopped' on a microtome. The wax dissolves completely in warm water and the section will then disintegrate. Tissues impregnated with water soluble wax are difficult to store as either blocks or sections since they are hygroscopic and will gradually dissolve away in the moisture present in the air and will begin to dissolve in the moisture from the skin if they are handled for more than a second or two. They must always be kept in a desiccator. For these reasons they have never become widely used.

Ester and polyester wax

These were introduced by Steedman and consist of ethylene glycol esters. They are based on glycol distearates.

Ester wax:

Diethylene glycol distearate	60%	
Polyethylene distearate (300)	10%	
Glyceryl monostearate	30%	

Polyester wax:

Polyethylene distearate (400)	90%
Cetyl alcohol	10%

Ester wax melts at 45–47°C whilst polyester wax melts at 38°C. Both are miscible with most dehydrating agents as well as clearing agents, so the amount of processing needed can be reduced. These waxes are extremely hard despite their low melting point and ester wax will even allow sectioning of small pieces of undecalcified bone. They do need to be kept dry since the waxes are slightly hygroscopic, but this is less of a problem than with the water soluble waxes. Sections can be briefly floated on to a cool water bath but must not be left floating for long or they will disintegrate.

Ester wax is probably the most popular and plays a small but still useful role in some areas of histology and histochemistry where its low melting point and hardness outweigh its extra problems and expense. Polyester wax has never been as popular as ester wax as it is more difficult to handle and blocks will even melt in a warm hand.

Celloidin and low viscosity nitrocellulose

This material is a derivative of cellulose and, although completely insoluble in water, it is soluble in a mixture of ethanol and diethyl ether. It is used in a different way to both wax and plastics by being used as a solution and then hardened by evaporating the solvent. This is a slow process and is very sensitive to the rate of evaporation.

The tissue is dehydrated in ethanol, treated with 1 : 1 ethanol and diethyl ether and then gradually infiltrated with a solution of celloidin in the same mixture. Depending on the formulation of the nitrocellulose it finally ends up with a concentration of 8–20% nitrocellulose. The tissue is then blocked out in a large mould with an excess of the mixture. This excess is needed because the celloidin shrinks a great deal as the solvent evaporates. The solvent is then evaporated slowly in an almost sealed container.

Rapid evaporation will harden the surface quickly but leave the centre of the block still liquid. Once solidified to the right texture the block can be fully hardened by exposure to chloroform vapour. The hardened block is then stored in alcohol. Storage in air results in the block becoming brittle as the remainder of the solvent evaporates.

The block can be attached to the microtome chuck using a thick celloidin solution or a commercial adhesive and the block can then be cut on a sliding microtome. Rotary microtomes are not used as the block needs to be kept moist and this needs a horizontal block face.

The block cuts well provided cutting is slow and the block and knife are kept moist with alcohol. Sections are stored in alcohol and are usually stained as free-floating sections rather than attached to slides. Sections need to be much thicker than with the other embedding media as celloidin is less rigid.

Celloidin is good for tissues with widely differing textures. I have found it useful for whole eyes where there is a tough outer coat around a soft inner material (the humours) and it is the only method which I have found that will reliably keep the retina attached.

Double embedding

In this technique the tissue is dehydrated and then impregnated with celloidin dissolved in methyl benzoate rather than the ether/alcohol used in the previous technique. The block is not allowed to

Celloidin or collodion is cellulose dinitrate and is a close relative of the explosive gun cotton. Although it is not explosive itself it is highly flammable. It was widely used as a plastic when it was usually mixed with camphor to form celluloid. It was used to make the backing material for the early cinema film. It is not stable when completely dry so many of these old 'nitrate' films are now falling apart. The solution was also used as a wound dressing by painting an alcoholic solution over wounds to give a clear protective covering ('Nuskin').

The decline in its commercial use has raised its price substantially as it is now a specialist chemical. It can be used for covering sections that are lifting, protecting micro-incinerated sections and coating crumbling blocks to enable sectioning. Although a valuable material for many tasks in histology it is unfortunately becoming too costly for routine use.

dry in this method and instead it is cleared in toluene and finally impregnated with molten paraffin wax. The tissue thus has a double support of celloidin and wax, and this may help with some difficult tissues but without the cutting and storage problems of full celloidin embedding. Double embedded blocks can be cut, stained and stored just like a paraffin block. It is a compromise and the heating that occurs when impregnating in the wax does lose some of the advantages of the cold celloidin technique but it is a worthwhile compromise and can be useful.

So the support of tissues can be achieved in a number of ways. Each has its own particular advantages and problems. The choice of technique is often critical in obtaining good sections, so it is important to know that alternatives are available. In routine histology the different methods are not used as extensively as they might be because paraffin wax impregnation is readily available and used every day. Many routine histologists will often just 'put up with' a paraffin block because it would be too much hassle to set up a different processing schedule for one block. In research or specialized laboratories, however, these alternative techniques are often still used and esteemed for their individual properties.

Suggested further reading

Anderson, G. and Gordon, K.C. (1996). Tissue processing, microtomy and paraffin sections, in *Theory and Practice of Histological Techniques* (eds J.D. Bancroft and A. Stevens). Edinburgh: Churchill Livingstone.

Culling, C.F.A. (1975). *Handbook of Histopathological and Histochemical Techniques*. London: Butterworths.

Self-assessment questions

1. What are the advantages of embedding in plastics?
2. Why are epoxy resins preferred for EM?
3. Why do epoxy resin sections not stain as well as wax or methacrylate sections?
4. Water soluble waxes (polyethylene glycols) support tissues well during cutting but are difficult to flatten. Why?
5. Give two advantages of ester wax and two disadvantages.
6. How does impregnating with celloidin differ from impregnating with wax?

Key Concepts and Facts

Plastic Embedding
- Plastics give firmer support than wax and allow thinner sections to be prepared.

- Processing for plastic embedding requires dehydration but clearing is not always needed.

- Plastics are hardened by polymerization and hardening is irreversible.

- Acrylic resins are useful for light microscopy but epoxy resins are preferred for electron microscopy.

Other Waxes
- Other waxy materials are occasionally used for embedding but are much less common.

Celloidin
- Celloidin is useful for some tough materials but thin sections are difficult.

Chapter 5
Cryotechniques

Learning objectives

After studying this chapter you should confidently be able to:

Outline the principles involved in the preparation of frozen sections.

Compare different methods of freezing tissues.

State the advantages of frozen sections compared to other embedding techniques.

Outline the process of freeze-drying.

The main use in hospitals for frozen sections is for the rapid diagnosis of tumours. Tumours can be benign (relatively innocuous) or malignant (the cancers) and the treatment of the two types can be very different. Benign tumours are removed with very little excess normal tissue but malignant tumours warrant a more extensive removal, including local lymph nodes.

Diagnosis from clinical examination of the patient is not always possible and a biopsy sample may be needed to confirm the diagnosis. The speed of the cryostat technique allows tissue to be frozen quickly, sectioned and stained ready for diagnosis within 15 min so the surgeon can decide the extent of the removal once a microscopic diagnosis is made. With modern anaesthetics it is safer to keep a patient anaesthetized for an extra quarter of an hour than to sew them back up, send them back to the ward and give them a second operation one or two days later. This limits the patient to one trip to the operating theatre instead of two and eliminates the worrying wait while the tissue is processed.

In the previous chapters on the main methods of preparing tissues it has been emphasized that in order to cut thin sections from soft human tissues such as liver or kidney the tissue needs a rigid support. The previous methods all involved removing the water from the tissues by treatment with dehydrating agents and then replacing it with wax or other hard materials. However, there is an alternative to this chemical replacement of the water in the tissues with a firm wax and that is to physically convert the water itself into a solid (ice) by lowering the temperature.

Cryotomy

Cryotomy is the term used to describe the use of ice as a support for section cutting. Freezing is quicker than replacement and does not involve treating the tissues with chemicals such as alcohol which may remove important materials (such as lipids) from the tissues or may alter the chemical properties of tissue components such as enzymes. Such techniques are usually called **frozen section techniques** and are an important way of preparing tissues for rapid diagnosis and for histochemistry.

There are several methods of cutting frozen sections but the most important difference between them concerns whether the microtome is entirely enclosed in a deep-freeze cabinet (usually at -15 to $-30°C$) or if the microtome is on a laboratory bench at room temperature with only the block being kept cold. In the most popular method the instrument involved, which consists of a deep freeze cabinet and the enclosed microtome, is called a **cryostat**.

Freezing and tissue damage

Freezing of tissues for frozen sections can damage the tissues and, although frozen sections involve less treatment of the tissues, there are still artefacts produced and these depend on how the tissue is frozen.

Slow freezing and mechanical damage

The rate of freezing alters the size of the ice crystals. At slow freezing rates the ice crystals will grow quite large and the crystals themselves expand as they freeze. This expansion results in mechanical damage to the tissue. Ice crystals may occur intracellularly and if they grow sufficiently large they can cause noticeable crevices in the tissue (ice crystal artefacts).

Water at atmospheric pressure is converted to ice at any temperature below $0°C$ but the ice crystals are in a dynamic state and will be constantly changing shape and interacting with adjacent ice crystals. Ice crystal damage gets worse as blocks are stored, as the ice remodels and changes its size and shape. Only when the temperature of the ice drops very low, about $-130°C$ for pure water, does it become stable and will not recrystallize. The point at which recrystallization in tissues, which are filled with a salt solution, is inhibited is not known but it is probably somewhere below $-90°C$. Storage of blocks must be done in liquid nitrogen at $-196°C$ to minimize this damage and cells should preferably be treated with a cryoprotectant solution such as 30% glycerol to reduce freezing damage.

Rapid freezing gives better tissue structure

Rapid freezing results in many smaller ice crystals that are less likely to cause visible alteration to the tissues. It follows that for high magnifications the ice crystals must be small enough not to cause visible damage. Rapid freezing is needed for high magnifications. For low magnifications or macroscopic examination (i.e. just using the unaided human eye) the rate of freezing can be slower since the slight ice crystal damage will not be seen. If the tissue is fixed before freezing it will be able to resist damage more easily, so slower freezing of fixed tissue is less damaging to the structure of the fixed tissue than similar freezing of fresh tissue.

Slow freezing and osmotic damage

The fluids in tissues are not pure water but a solution of various salts, so when freezing occurs it is the effects on a salt solution that

Although fast freezing is best for tissue structure it is actually much more dangerous to living tissues that are not protected. In slow freezing most of the ice crystals form outside the cells and are made of pure ice. This increases the osmotic pressure of the fluid since the same amount of salt is now dissolved in a smaller volume. The cells shrink as they lose fluid to the extracellular spaces but there is no necrosis (necrosis is where cells are killed). Fast freezing freezes the cell cytoplasm as well as the extracellular tissues and this is intensely necrotizing.

The freezing effect is not the cause of the necrosis seen in cold injury such as frost-bite and trench foot. These injuries are caused by the capillaries in the area constricting and reducing oxygenation of the tissues. Ischaemic damage results and this can cause the loss of fingers and toes.

need to be considered not simply the effects on water. Slow freezing of a salt solution results in the production of ice crystals that are pure water. It is only when the temperature gets below $-21°C$ that the tissue fluid will freeze as a whole. Since water is being removed from the cellular fluid the remaining solution becomes more concentrated. Water will be drawn out from the cells and they will shrink as a result.

Depression of freezing point

Salts dissolved in water lower the freezing point of the solution (depression of freezing point) and a temperature of $-10°C$ is required before tissue fluid will freeze. The liquid left behind as the water crystallizes as pure ice may eventually become so concentrated that even at very low temperatures it may not freeze. The unfrozen areas will therefore remain liquid and the tissues in these regions will be unsupported. The result is that these areas will not section well and the sections may have distinctive holes where the pools of unfrozen tissue fluid occurred. The tissue appears to have holes in it and this can make it look like a waffle and this artefact has been called **waffle artefact**. The production of this artefact is dependent on the rate of cooling. If the rate of freezing is high enough then the tissue freezes as one intact block without separating into water and salt solution.

Rate of cooling and heat conduction

The rate at which tissues freeze depends on conduction from the warmer tissues to the coolant. The rate of conduction is dependent on the temperature difference between the coolant and the tissue, so the lower the temperature of the coolant the faster the tissue freezes. So even though the tissue may need to be cut at $-20°C$ it is usual to cool it with a cooling system that will be at a much lower temperature and then allow the block to warm up to the cutting temperature. This means that the tissue reaches $-20°C$ much quicker and so there is less deterioration.

Conduction and area in contact with the coolant

The rate of freezing is also dependent on the area in contact with the coolant. With a solid coolant packed around the microtome chuck or a Peltier module the only contact is with the base of the block. Cooling will spread through the tissues from the base and this can be seen as a white line moving up the block. Cooling will be slightly slower at the top of the block since the heat has to transfer through the block as well as through the chuck. Anything that slows down the transfer of heat will similarly slow down the rate of freezing. Microtome chucks should therefore be made of

The effects of freezing can be seen in frozen strawberries that retain their flavour but lose their texture. The firmness of strawberries is due to turgor pressure. This is a higher pressure inside the cell pressing against the cellulose cell wall like an inner-tube in a bicycle tyre. When frozen the ice crystals rupture the cell membrane. The cell deflates like a punctured tyre and the strawberry loses its firm texture. Chemically it is unchanged but its physical integrity is lost.

Freezing human tissue to keep it alive is not easy and requires replacement of the normal tissue fluid with cryopreservative and controlled freezing. The people who have paid thousands of pounds to have their bodies cryogenically stored are unlikely to be able to be restored even with advancing technology since all their cells are likely to be damaged and repairing punctures in every cell in the body is totally impractical.

metal and putting thick layers of insulating materials such as cork on top of the chuck should be avoided.

With liquid coolants the whole block can be immersed in the coolant and this increases the surface area for heat transfer and can speed up cooling. The disadvantage is that the fluid may itself damage the block. Liquid coolants can, of course, also be used to simply cool the chuck without totally immersing the specimen.

Methods of cooling tissues for sectioning

Various techniques have been employed to reduce the temperature of the tissues below freezing.

Slow freezing methods

Slow freezing is taken here to mean a freezing technique in which it takes several minutes to freeze the tissue into a solid block and which will produce larger crystals that may give damage that is visible with high magnifications.

Freezing tissues in a deep-freeze cabinet

Simply putting the tissue into a deep-freeze cabinet at -20 to $-30°C$ will eventually freeze the tissues. This is usually done histologically by putting the tissue into the chamber of a cryostat which is normally held at $-20°C$. Some cryostats have an extra-cold shelf or chamber that may be as low as $-40°C$ which freezes the tissue more rapidly, but it is still a relatively slow process. The use of a deep freeze or a cryostat is a cheap and easy method of freezing tissues since it involves no special reagents or even extra equipment. It is, however, very slow and may take hours for anything other than very small blocks. This very slow freezing causes quite a lot of damage and is only suitable for macroscopic work such as whole body autoradiography. Even quite low magnifications will reveal some damage from the frozen ice crystals.

Freezing tissues with a thermoelectric module

Peltier modules or thermoelectric modules utilize the fact that when current is passed across two different conductors they absorb heat on one side and emit it on the other surface. By stacking several thermoelectric modules together an efficient heat removal can be achieved. The two materials most commonly used in the thermo-electric modules are bismuth telluride and copper. Thermoelectric modules act as 'heat pumps' and move the heat from the specimen and pump it into a heat sink. The usual heat sink is a current of water which is used to cool the underside of the module. The rate at

Cooling is not only a problem for the histologist but is also needed in electronics. Peltier modules are now used to transfer heat away from heat-producing electronic devices such as microprocessors, since once they overheat they stop working. The sprays used for cooling tissues are also used to cool electronic circuits. It is an easy way to find a failing device. When a component starts to fail it will often work for a short while after switching on and then fail once it overheats. By spraying one circuit component at a time and seeing when the instrument starts working again you then know that you have just sprayed the failing part of the circuit.

The sprays are also used by plumbers when it is not possible to turn off a water supply to replace a stopcock or tap. The pipe leading to the stopcock is sprayed until there is solid ice inside. The stopcock can then be replaced quickly before the ice melts.

which heat is extracted is controlled by the strength of the electric current. Increasing the current means a faster rate of freezing.

The tissue will eventually reach an equilibrium where the rate of heat extraction is the same as the rate of heat gain. Since heat gain from the environment is dependent on the temperature difference between the tissue and the environment, the faster the heat is removed the lower the equilibrium temperature will be. Since the rate of heat pumping depends on the current it means that the temperature of the block can be easily controlled by altering the current.

Thermoelectric modules provide a very convenient way of freezing tissue and are cheap to run and extremely controllable. One of the commonest ways of using these modules is to incorporate them as the chuck of the microtome and simply freeze the tissue on to the Peltier module on the microtome. The modules require a supply of water and electricity, so the associated wires and pipes usually make them a little bit unwieldy for use directly on microtomes where the block moves and the knife stays still but they are easily attached to microtomes where the knife movement provides the cutting action and the block remains relatively still. The reversal of the current is a convenient way to melt the lower surface of the block and allow it to be removed.

Rapid freezing methods

Rapid freezing techniques are now the most popular methods and which one is preferred is often a matter of availability rather than strict scientific choice. Most of these methods will give excellent results if carefully done.

Freezing using a fast-evaporating liquid

This involves commercial spray cans containing fast-evaporating liquids (e.g. dichlorodifluoromethane or the ozone friendlier chlorofluorocarbons). As a liquid evaporates it will absorb heat which is called the latent heat of evaporation. This property applies to all liquids but the faster they evaporate the faster they absorb heat. The liquids chosen for these sprays will evaporate very quickly and therefore absorb heat very quickly. They tend to be expensive to use on a regular basis when compared to other methods of freezing and typically achieve a temperature of about $-50°C$.

They are very convenient since they can be easily transported and are therefore available to freeze tissue in places a long way from the laboratory. The sprays are a good reserve or emergency method of freezing as they can be kept in store without deteriorating. They can damage the outside of the block if they are sprayed directly on to the specimen because they are initially liquid and therefore act as solvents, but they do not penetrate beyond the very edge of the block so the inner regions are not affected.

Fast-evaporating liquids are also the method of cooling in some 'self-cooling' drinks. These are cans of drink with a widget incorporated into them which releases a fast-evaporating liquid and this drops the temperature of the can by $15°C$ in $90s$. The advantages are obvious but the dangers are also great. The coolant (HFC134a, 1,1,1,2-tetrafluoroethane) is not a risk to the ozone layer so it is not banned by the Montreal Convention but is a powerful greenhouse gas, causing over 3000 times more global warming than carbon dioxide. If such cans go on sale and become a success then the amounts released could totally outweigh all the efforts to reduce carbon dioxide emissions. At the time of writing the British Government and the EU are considering banning these cans.

The use of these materials in laboratories is more defensible since much smaller amounts are used and they are used for diagnosing life-threatening disease. This means that the risk–benefit analysis is quite different, but whenever a product is being used the impact on the environment must be considered.

Cooling with carbon dioxide

This method of cooling relies on the sudden expansion of high pressure liquid CO_2 from a cylinder. It rapidly expands to a gas and absorbs heat in the expansion phase. The same effect is seen with CO_2 fire extinguishers which produce a jet that appears white because of the production of cold CO_2 snow. Also like the fire extinguishers, CO_2 cooling is very noisy. When the CO_2 is released it expands rapidly causing a very loud hissing noise.

CO_2 cylinders are reasonably convenient in the laboratory where they are only occasionally moved but are more difficult to transport to distant sites. CO_2 cylinders are quite reasonably priced and are readily available since they are also used for pumping (for example beer in pubs). The cylinders must be used so that they run the liquid CO_2 out of the cylinder and not just the gas. This requires either a special siphoned cylinder which can be used upright or an ordinary one can be used inverted (outlet at the bottom). CO_2 blasts can reach temperatures down to $-70°C$.

Cooling using solid carbon dioxide

Solid carbon dioxide is also called 'cardice' or dry ice. This can be bought as large blocks and can also be prepared from liquid CO_2 by trapping the CO_2 snow produced when the liquid expands. The solid CO_2 can be used as a dry material by packing it around the microtome chuck to cool it. Alternatively the solid CO_2 can be mixed with acetone to produce a freezing mixture in which chucks or tissues can be immersed. Both methods achieve a temperature of about $-70°C$. Buying blocks of CO_2 can be quite expensive and inconvenient as solid carbon dioxide must be delivered daily.

Cooling with liquid nitrogen

This liquefied gas is very cold ($-196°C$). Liquid nitrogen can be cheap if produced on site or bought in bulk. The very low temperature gives the possibility of very rapid freezing but there are some problems.

Liquid nitrogen has a tendency to boil when it comes in contact with warmer objects. The mechanical effects of boiling may damage some delicate tissues and the boiling slows down the rate of freezing. This slowing is due to the boiling at the surface of the block producing a layer of nitrogen gas around the block which acts as a layer of insulation and inhibits the transfer of heat.

To get around this problem various techniques are used. Some workers simply use liquid nitrogen to cool less volatile liquids such as isopentane which do not boil and then use the cooled isopentane to cool the actual block. The isopentane becomes quite viscous at these low temperatures and the viscosity is used as an indication of when the cooling has reached the correct temperature. Other

Although liquid nitrogen is very cold it is still reasonably safe because of the boiling effect, and the liquid nitrogen will simply run off anything warm like skin with the drops of liquid nitrogen held aloft like a miniature hovercraft on a cushion of nitrogen gas. It is a party trick of some conjurors and exhibitionists to pour liquid nitrogen on their hands. This is not my idea of a safe trick and liquid nitrogen does become extremely dangerous if it becomes trapped and cannot roll away. So folds in skin or clothing become dangerous traps for the supercold liquid. If treated with caution it is safe but mishandled it can be a disaster.

workers use metal foil to enhance the rate of cooling. The speed of cooling can also be improved by using powdered starch ('glove powder') in the form of a dusting on the surface of the block. The fine powder reduces the boiling effect in the same way as boiling beads do in a beaker of heated liquid.

Rather than cooling a liquid the liquid nitrogen can be used to cool large-blade metal forceps which are then applied to the tissue. This technique can be used to freeze tissues whilst they are still in the body to eliminate the time between removal and freezing. It only works well with very small pieces of tissue and special forceps which have extra-heavy jaws which act as large heat sinks to draw the heat out of the tissue without themselves becoming warmed significantly.

Cutting sections using a freezing microtome

The freezing microtome technique uses a microtome with some convenient method of freezing the tissue on to the chuck (e.g. a carbon dioxide blast or Peltier module) but only the specimen is kept cold. The rest of the microtome and the air around the microtome are at room temperature.

Tissue should be fixed first

The tissue usually needs to be fixed in formaldehyde to harden it and enable thin sections to be cut since it is common for the sections to thaw out during the cutting process. Fixation in formaldehyde is best as it does not interfere with the freezing process and leaves the tissue fairly flexible. Mercury-, chromium- or osmium-based fixatives overharden the tissues, making thin sectioning difficult, and the salts can depress the freezing point of the tissue. Alcohol-based fixatives will not freeze since the freezing point of alcohol is very low ($-112°C$). Unfixed sections can be cut using a freezing microtome but they will often disintegrate during sectioning or staining.

The tissue is frozen on to the chuck

Tissue can be attached to the microtome chuck using simply water or saline as an adhesive though some workers prefer to use a gum syrup that has a thicker consistency. A piece of filter-paper soaked in water placed on top of the chuck is often useful as it makes it easier to remove the tissue cleanly after sectioning.

Tissue can be frozen solid by one of the methods discussed previously, with the thermoelectric module and CO_2 blast being the most common. Once frozen they are cut using a conventional microtome and knife, usually a non-disposable knife since ice is somewhat harder than wax.

Collection of free-floating sections

If the sections are cut very quickly they can be made to jump off the knife directly into a bath of fluid but this is difficult to control. If the sections are cut more slowly then sections melt on the knife and can be removed using a brush moistened with water. Although it is possible to attach the sections on to a slide and then air dry them to achieve adhesion they are usually easily washed off even when using an adhesive such as gelatine. More often the sections are left free-floating and transferred from one reagent to another by draping it over a bent glass rod ('glass hockey stick'). This is more difficult than using a section attached to a slide and the final stained section still needs to be attached to a slide before mounting under a coverslip.

Cold knife technique

The section can be prevented from melting by cooling the knife and this also helps to reduce crumpling. The knife can be cooled by using solid carbon dioxide held on to the knife or by repeatedly blasting the knife with carbon dioxide or even by clamping a Peltier module to the knife. The ideal is to keep the knife well below freezing at between -10 and $-20°C$. The sections still have a tendency to roll and must be teased out during cutting using a fine brush. In the full cold knife technique the tissues are placed on to a slide and into fixative before thawing occurs. This is difficult in practice and most workers simply use a cooled knife to give better sections.

Although widely used at one time all the freezing microtome techniques are now uncommon for most tissues, but are used more in neurological histology.

Cryostats

The cryostat or cold microtome technique involves keeping all the parts of the cutting at low temperature. The block, the microtome knife and indeed the whole microtome as well as the final section are kept below freezing. The cryostat is therefore a specially designed deep-freeze cabinet into which a microtome fits and with connections to allow the common controls to be operated from outside the cabinet without the microtomist having to put his hands into the cold chamber. This not only keeps the operators hands warm but also stops the cabinet temperature from rising too much. A light is usually fitted inside so that it is easy to see what is happening on the microtome. There is usually a transparent lid to allow viewing while still keeping the chamber cold. There is also usually an antimisting system and an automatic defrost system.

The freezing microtome has often been more popular with neurohistologists than with routine histologists. It is often quicker and simpler to cut large blocks of brain with a large freezing microtome than it is to process them through to other embedding media. The thicker sectioning associated with the freezing microtome is not a major problem. The sections needed for many neurological methods are often much thicker than for the rest of the body since the intention is to follow the nerve cell processes. Free-floating sections are always more difficult to handle than ones attached to the slide but have the advantage of presenting two surfaces from which the dyes and reagents can penetrate.

Good quality sections from unfixed tissues

Sections produced in the cryostat are generally of a much better quality than those from the freezing microtome. In the cryostat even unfixed tissue will section well. In fact fresh tissue generally cuts better and is easier to handle than fixed tissue. It is much more usual to fix after cutting than before and, since the section always remains frozen, there is no need to thaw the sections which can be fixed while still frozen. It is also very common not to fix the tissues until after staining. Unfixed tissues are widely used in histochemistry. Variations on this technique are the most common methods for preparing frozen sections.

Freezing is done outside the cryostat

Tissues are usually attached to the microtome chuck outside the cryostat and then quickly transferred into the cold chamber of the cryostat. The attachment to the microtome chuck is fairly straight-forward. The metal microtome chuck has a piece of moist filterpaper placed on top and the fresh tissue is placed on top of this and the chuck and tissue are frozen by one of the rapid freezing techniques.

Tissues can be supported

If it is difficult to keep the tissue in position it can be surrounded and supported by a gum solution or one of the commercial products (OCT or Cryo-m-bed) which contain polyvinyl derivatives which are inert, water soluble and colourless. These are thick, viscous solutions that allow awkward-shaped pieces of tissue to be temporarily held in place whilst freezing occurs. Once frozen these support media cut smoothly and evenly with a similar texture to soft tissues.

Cutting cryostat sections

The microtome fitted into the cryostat can be of any type, but sliding and complex rotary microtomes can be difficult to lubricate at such low temperatures so modified rocking microtomes are often fitted instead. Sections cut at low temperature have a tendency to roll up and most cryostats use an antiroll plate to keep them flat. This is simply a transparent plate of perspex arranged in such a way that it leaves a narrow gap between the plate and the knife. This gap is wide enough to allow the section to slide down but narrow enough to prevent rolling. The correct adjustment of the antiroll plate is one of the most important factors in producing good sections. The antiroll plate is also one of the reasons why even laboratories that regularly use disposable knives for their wax sectioning still use solid non-disposable knives in the cryostat. It

role in the selectivity of dyes but are usually secondary to ionic bonds unless special conditions are arranged to inhibit ionic interactions. This inhibition of ionic bonds can be achieved by using a non-aqueous solvent (water inhibits hydrogen bonding and favours ionization), high salt concentration (which competes with the dye for tissue ion binding sites) and extreme pH (which is chosen to inhibit the ionization of tissue groups).

One or two instances of staining involve hydrogen bonding rather than ionic bonding. In the staining of elastin fibres hydrogen bonds are probably more important than ionic forces. More controversially, the staining of amyloid by Congo red has been considered to be dominated by hydrogen bond staining.

Van der Waals forces

These are short range forces and will only have an effect if the two atoms are between about 0.12 and 0.2 nm apart. If they are further apart then there is no effective bonding force. These van der Waals forces can occur between any two atoms and are not specific for any atom or group. If the surface shape of the tissue protein and the shape of the dye match then many van der Waals bonds can be formed. So, although they are individually very weak, they may add up to a significant binding force if the dye and protein have exactly complementary molecular surfaces (Figure 6.6). The van der Waals forces are believed to have a role in selectivity but probably only play a minor role in attracting the dye to the tissue.

The ability to form many van der Waals bonds is one explanation of the finding that larger dyes will bind more strongly than small dyes even though they have no more ionizable groups. Van der Waals bonds are unaffected by pH, ions and hydrogen bonding agents.

Covalent bonds

These are very strong bonds and are not easily broken once formed. They do not seem to be important in most staining reactions. They are important in some histochemical techniques, e.g. periodic acid

Van der Waals forces are probably important in staining but in a quite different way to the binding of the dye. The adhesion of the section to the slide involves van der Waals interactions between the section and the glass. As the water evaporates from under the section the whole undersurface of the section comes in contact with the flat, smooth surface of the slide. Millions of interactions are caused and the section is then firmly adherent.

With the use of silane-treated slides there is the addition of charge to the surface, and the increased strength of adhesion may well reflect the difference in strength of the two bonds.

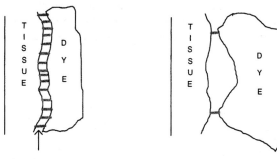

Van der Waals bonds

Figure 6.6 *Van der Waals forces and dye binding. The dye and tissue on the left have similar shapes so every atom in the structures can be brought close enough to form van der Waals forces. This large number of weak bonds will be a significant binding force. On the right the dye is not complementary in shape so only a few atoms will be close enough to form bonds. The dye on the right will be less strongly bound and will be displaced more easily than the dye on the left*

Schiff staining and in the attachment of dyes to antibodies in immunofluorescence. The so-called **reactive dyes** use covalent bonds to bind but are not used much in histology.

Hydrophobic interactions

Although they are sometimes called hydrophobic bonds the forces involved are not chemical bonds in the conventional sense since these hold dyes in tissues by the exclusion of water from the regions of hydrophobic groups. The exclusion of water stabilizes the two groups involved by entropy/enthalpy changes. Hydrophobic interactions are again short range and are unaffected by hydrogen bonding agents or salts. Altering the pH may, however, change a particular group from a hydrophilic to a hydrophobic form by altering its ionization and this will alter the staining with hydrophobic dyes. Hydrophobic interactions are important in selectivity and play a major role in the staining of lipids.

Dye structure

Dyes are coloured organic compounds that can selectively bind to tissues. Most modern dyes are synthesized from simpler organic molecules, usually benzene or one of its derivatives. The modification of these compounds into dyes is a huge industry and the chemistry of dye synthesis can be complex, but a simple example will show the general nature of dye structure.

Chromophores

Most simple organic compounds such as alkanes, benzene and alcohols are colourless to the human eye but will absorb light outside the visible spectrum. Benzene for example absorbs strongly in the ultraviolet region of the spectrum but appears water-white to the human eye. The benzene must be altered so that it will absorb visible light and so become a visibly coloured compound that can be useful as a dye. Any group that makes an organic compound coloured is called a **chromophore**. Benzene can be made to absorb visible light by adding a suitable chromophore. In the example given in Figure 6.7 the chromophore used is the nitro group. Adding a single nitro group gives nitrobenzene which is a pale yellow colour, adding a second and third group intensifies the yellow colour and trinitrobenzene is a strong yellow colour.

Auxochromes

Trinitrobenzene, although coloured, is still not a dye as it will not bind to tissues. Treating the section with trinitrobenzene will temporarily colour it yellow in the same way that a plastic

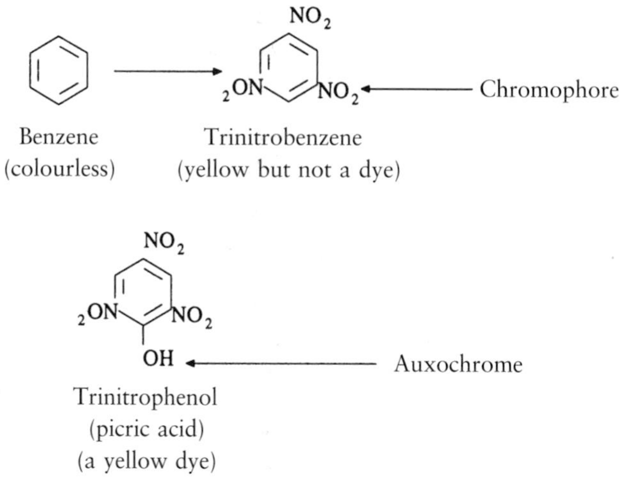

Benzene
(colourless)

Trinitrobenzene
(yellow but not a dye)

———————— Chromophore

Trinitrophenol
(picric acid)
(a yellow dye)

———————— Auxochrome

Figure 6.7 *The conversion of benzene into a dye by the addition of a chromophore and auxochrome*

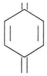

Figure 6.8 *Quininoid structure, illustrating an important chromophore*

sponge appears coloured when it is soaked in a coloured liquid, but the colour will wash out as soon as the tissue is rinsed in a solvent. To turn a coloured compound into a dye requires the addition of an ionizable group that will enable the dye to bind to the tissues. Such binding groups are called **auxochromes**. The addition of an ionizable OH group turns trinitrobenzene into the dye trinitrophenol, which is more commonly called picric acid in histology. Picric acid is an acid dye (the OH group is phenolic and ionizes by losing a hydrogen ion) and is very useful in histology and is an essential part of the popular van Gieson counterstain.

The most important chromophoric group in dye structure is not the nitro group but the quininoid arrangement of the benzene ring (Figure 6.8). This has two double bonds at either end of the ring and two double bonds on either side. This arrangement strongly absorbs parts of the visible light spectrum.

Changing substituent groups

The exact colour of a dye is very dependent on many other features of the molecule including molecular size and other substituents on the ring. Most auxochromes alter the colour of the dye slightly (hence their name) as well as allowing the dye to bind to the tissues. Other groups or atoms are introduced solely to alter the colour and these are called modifier groups. Modifiers do not greatly alter the staining characteristics of the molecule, they simply alter the shade of colour.

Trivial names of dyes

Dyes are mainly produced for industrial uses such as textile dyeing so a wide variety of different dyes have been synthesized to give a large range of colours. Dye manufacturers usually give the dyes

Picric acid is a powerful explosive and needs to be kept moist. It was known as Lyddite after the explosive works at Lydd where it was manufactured. It was originally discovered by oxidizing indigo, a natural dye from an Asiatic plant. Picric acid is an unusual material in histological terms since it is a good fixative and forms the basis of Bouin's fixative, and it is also a useful dye as it has a low molecular weight. It is also used in histochemical tests to dissolve and thus identify the pigments found in malarial cells and following formalin fixation.

Until the discovery of synthetic dyes by W.H. Perkin in the 19th century the only dyes available were natural dyes. These tended to be somewhat drab and they faded easily. The dye Tyrian purple was therefore a major discovery. Legend has it that this dye was discovered by the demigod Hercules. It is extracted from molluscs and by ancient standards was bright and did not fade quickly. It became a symbol of power and wealth in the ancient world and the dictionary still lists purple as representing wealth and power. The discovery of the first synthetic mauve dye was entirely accidental. W.H. Perkin was a chemistry student trying to make the drug quinine from coal tar when he found some bright purple crystals. He borrowed some money to set up a factory and established a synthetic dye industry – and was rich enough to retire at 35.

they produce trivial names such as eosin or Congo red rather than their full chemical names and some of these names are copyrighted.

The dye structure shown in Figure 6.9 illustrates the complexity of many of these dyes. The full chemical name of this structure is 3,3'-[[biphenyl]-4,4'-diylbis(azo)]-bis[4-amino-1-naphthalenesulphonic acid] disodium salt, whilst its trivial name is Congo red. The trivial name is easier to remember and to say so most histologists stick to the trivial names.

Different firms may have different names for the same compound and this can be very confusing. If you ask for a dye by one name and get a bottle back with a different name on the label you tend to think there has been a mistake. But if you order trypan blue you could get a bottle called chlorazol blue which is the same dye by a different name. Eosin Y (yellowish eosin) has the following alternative names: acid red 87, bromoacid J, bromoacid S, bromoacid TS, bromoacid XL, bromoacid XX, bromofluorescein and bronze bromo.

That a dye may have more than one name is bad enough but it is usually easy to check with the supplier who will be able to put your mind at rest. More of a problem is that different dyes can be sold by different manufacturers with the same name. For example a dye called light green is usually considered as an acid dye in histology and is used for staining connective tissue, but the term light green is also used by some manufacturers for some basic dyes which will stain the nucleus and not the connective tissues. Buying the wrong dye can totally alter the results of a staining method.

The trivial dye names are applied to their industrial use rather than their histological use, e.g. fast green FCF (for colouring food) and Brown FK (for kippers). In industrial terms an acid dye is one that would be used from an acidic solution and not necessarily one that would be anionic. Sometimes the names coincide with histological properties, e.g. basic fuchsin is a basic dye, but sometimes they are misleading, e.g. neutral red is a basic dye in histological terminology.

The Colour Index

To overcome all the confusion there is a standard list of all dyes, their synonyms and their structures. This is called the Colour Index. This is a monumental work of reference produced by **the Society of Dyers and Colourists** and each dye is given an individual number and then listed along with its name(s) and properties. Since

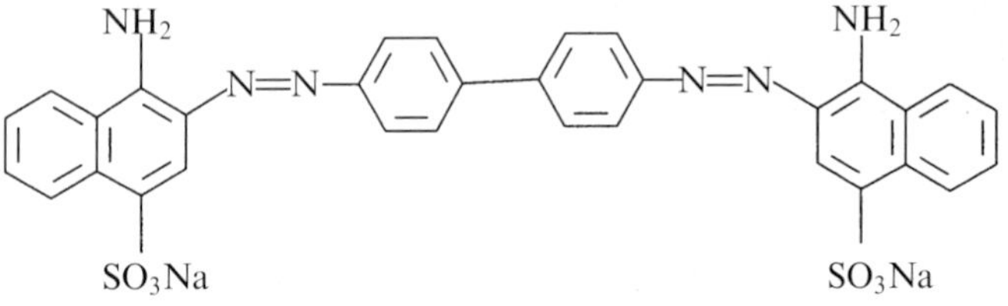

Figure 6.9 *Structure of Congo red*

each dye on the list has a unique number that identifies it, this list is the most reliable way to identify a dye. When naming a dye in techniques the CI number should be given to avoid ambiguity, e.g. eosin Y (CI 45380).

The numbers in the CI are arranged according to their structure with the most important feature being their chromophoric group. For example all nitroso dyes have numbers between 10000 and 10299, nitro dyes have numbers between 10300 and 10999, monoazo dyes have numbers between 11000 and 19999 and so on. There are 31 groups in all with CI numbers up to 78000. Not all of these groups include important histological dyes but a few of the more important groups are listed below with examples of histological dyes from the group.

1. **Nitro dyes.** These have the nitro group, $-NO_2$, as the chromophore, e.g. picric acid, martius yellow.
2. **Azo dyes.** These have the -N=N- group (azo) as the chromophore, e.g. orange G.
3. **Triaryl methane dyes.** These include the quininoid arrangement as the actual chromophore. The quininoid ring is shown as the one on the left in the diagram below but since all three benzene rings are equivalent there can be rearrangement of the bonds and any of the benzene rings could take up this arrangement. There are a great number of dyes used in histology that fall into this category and a few examples are methyl violet, methyl blue and aniline blue.

4. **Anthraquinone.** Here the quininoid ring is seen as the middle of the three fused rings. Examples are alizarin and carmine.

5. **Xanthene.** Here the quininoid ring is the right hand one of the three fused rings and the ring is tilted compared to the previous example. Examples include eosin and xanthene.

6. **Thiazine.** Very similar to the previous example in overall structure but the middle ring now has S and N as constituent atoms. This group contains many important metachromatic dyes, e.g. toluidine blue, methylene blue, azure A.

Histological classification

In histology it is often more useful to classify dyes by their action on tissues and hence their uses in histology. Two dyes within the same chemical group may have quite different uses in histology. For example the two anthraquinone dyes in the list above are used quite differently. Carmine is an important nuclear stain whilst alizarin is most commonly used to detect calcium in tissues. Also dyes that are from totally different groups may be quite easily exchanged in histological techniques. The histological classification is only a broad guide to how a dye will work in practice since the actual binding relies on many properties and not just the simple ionic nature.

Basic dyes are cationic and will stain anionic or acidic materials such as carboxylates, sulphates (many complex carbohydrates are sulphated) and phosphates (particularly the phosphates in nucleic acids). Most basic dyes are used as nuclear stains and staining of cytoplasmic carboxyl groups is deliberately suppressed by using a slightly acid pH. Acidic materials that stain with basic dyes are termed **basophilic**.

Acidic dyes are anionic and will stain cationic or basic groups in tissue such as amino groups. Most are used to stain proteins in the cytoplasm and connective tissues. Materials that stain with acid dyes are called **acidophilic**.

Neutral dyes are simply compounds of basic and acid dyes, e.g. by combining eosin and methylene blue the neutral dye methylene blue eosinate is formed. In this case both ions are coloured. Such dye complexes will stain both nucleus and cytoplasm from a single dye bath. Some neutral dyes called Romanowsky stains and are made from more complex mixtures. The Romanowsky dyes are the commonest dyes used in haematology (they are less common in histology but still very useful) and include Giemsa, Leishman and Wright's stains.

Amphoteric dyes also have both anionic and cationic groups but these are on the same ion. Such dyes can stain either the nucleus or the cytoplasm if conditions are appropriate.

Leuco compounds are dyes that have been rendered colourless by destroying their chromophores. They can be recolorized by tissues and are sometimes useful in histochemistry. Leuco patent blue has been used as a reagent to stain for haemoglobin peroxidase. Usually the chromophore is a quininoid ring and reduction will result in the loss of the quininoid arrangement and so the colour is lost.

Natural dyes are simply dye substances extracted from natural sources. Although the main source of dyes for early microscopists, they have largely been replaced by synthetic dyes (also sometimes called aniline dyes or coal tar dyes after the main starting materials) which are usually more reliable, cheaper and can be supplied more readily. Natural dyes still in use include haematoxylin, carmine, orcein and litmus, although synthetic varieties are also available for some of these.

Non-dye constituents of staining solutions

As well as dyes most staining solutions contain other materials to improve the staining. Acids are often added to alter the pH and acetic acid is probably the most popular acid used in this way. The solutions can be buffered for more precise pH control but this is unusual in histology though frequent in histochemistry.

Mordants

Mordanting is the use of a non-dyeing compound to improve the binding of the dye, with the mordant involved being able to mediate a dye–tissue interaction. Mordanting of dyes has a long history and was crucial in early textile dyeing to fix the stain to the fabric and make it into a fast dye. Fast in this sense does not mean rapid but resistant to washing out or fading; both of these properties are critical in the dyeing of textiles. However, the term mordant was very vague in its original usage and covered a number of mechanisms of binding dyes. The term has been adopted for some histological staining but its use in histology is more restricted. It is usually only applied to conditions where the mordant acts as a link between the dye and the tissue and where the mordant is a metal salt (Figure 6.10).

The mechanism by which the mordant binds to the tissues is not certain but one likely mechanism is a dative covalency. The link to the dye would involve more than one such dative bond, resulting in a chelate that is stable. The dye and mordant complex is called a **dye lake**. The groups on the dye forming the dative bonds are mainly oxygen-containing (e.g. in phenols, carboxyls and quinones) or nitrogen (in amine, azo and nitro groups).

Since it is the mordant that binds to the tissue the selectivity of the dye is controlled by selecting the mordant not the dye. The mordant gives greater stability to the stain and it is not easily removed by water, alcohols or weak acids (i.e. it is a fast dye) and this makes it ideal when other stains are to be used afterwards as the stain resists decolorization by the later reagents. Staining is commonly done

The dye woad was extracted from the leaves of *Isatis tinctoria* and was identical to indigo. The importation of indigo was strongly resisted by the dyers in Britain and the last woad mills closed only in the 1930s in Lincolnshire. This despite woad processing having the reputation of being the smelliest of industrial processes.

The methods used to make natural dyes stable and resistant to washing were often quite elaborate. Alums were commonly used as mordants so their transfer to histology is hardly surprising. Organic materials were also used including tannins from wood bark, gallic acids from tree galls and ammonia from urine.

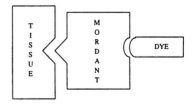

Figure 6.10 *Mordanting. The dye can only bind strongly to the tissue when the mordant acts as a link between the two*

The way in which dyes are used can differ. One distinction is between progressive and regressive staining. **Progressive staining** is the simplest form with the dye being applied to the section until the desired density of colour is reached. **Regressive staining** involves overstaining the tissue so it is darker than is needed and then removing the excess to bring the colour down to the required level. The removal of the excess dye is termed **differentiation**.

Regressive staining is often a better method of using stains. The reason is that dyes are rarely specific and will not only stain the structure being demonstrated but will also slightly colour the background albeit lighter than the object. By removing some dye the background can be cleared since the binding is usually less strong, so the dye will be removed quickly from the background. Provided that the object being viewed has more dye than is required, the differentiation will simply bring the colour down to the optimal level.

with the dye and mordant being present in the same solution, thus forming the dye lake in the stain before being applied to the tissues (e.g. Harris's haematoxylin and carmalum). The dye and the mordant can also be used in two separate steps (e.g. Heidenhain's haematoxylin) and one or two techniques have used post-mordanting in which the dye is applied first and the mordant added afterwards.

Regressive use of mordants

It is also common to use mordanted dyes **regressively** (see Box). The differentiation is done by using strong acids (e.g. hydrochloric acid often in alcoholic solution). Differentiation can also be done using excess mordant, for example the iron alum in Heidenhain's haematoxylin can be used to slowly remove the excess haematoxylin. The excess mordant acts by displacing the dye lake and replacing it with a mordant with no attached dye. Theoretically it should be possible to devise a stain in which the balance of mordant to dye gives self-differentiation. A self-differentiating haematoxylin was published by Baker but requires a constant and reliable dye that is generally not available since most mordanting is done with natural dyes that vary in their composition from one year to the next.

Trapping agents

These differ from mordants in that they are always applied after the dye. They form large aggregates with the dye and result in the dye precipitating in the tissue. The large precipitate is more difficult to remove and resists differentiation. The best known example is the use of iodine to trap the violet dye inside the relatively impermeable wall of Gram-positive bacteria whilst it can be removed from the more permeable Gram-negative organisms.

Accentuators and accelerators

Accentuators and accelerators are materials added to staining solutions to improve the staining reaction. Accentuators are generally simply methods of controlling pH, e.g. potassium hydroxide in Loeffler's methylene blue and phenol in carbol fuchsin. Accelerators are found in neurological techniques and are often hypnotic drugs such as barbiturates or chloral hydrate but the mechanism of this enhancement is not known.

Metachromatic dyes and metachromasia

The term metachromasia is used when a dye stains a tissue component a different colour to the dye solution. For example toluidine blue is a strong basic blue dye that stains nuclei a deep blue colour; however, it will also stain mast cell granules a pink colour. This colour shift with mast cells is **metachromasia** whilst the usual blue staining is called orthochromasia. Many dyes can show metachromasia but the thiazine group dyes are especially good for this type of staining. Metachromasia is important as it is highly selective and only certain tissue structures can stain metachromatically. Materials that can be stained in this way are called chromotropes and they include mucins, especially the sulphated mucins, and mast cell granules.

Mechanism of colour shift in metachromasia

The colour shift in metachromasia is always from a blue or violet dye to yellow or red staining. This means that the colour absorption shifts to shorter wavelengths, leaving only the longer wavelengths to be seen. This is believed to represent a polymerization of the dye. The greater the degree of polymerization the stronger the metachromasia. For example, toluidine blue will stain hyaluronic acid a blue colour, pectic acid (found in plants) a purple and mast cell granules a definite red colour. The difference is in the spacing of the acid groups as shown in Table 6.1 and Figure 6.11.

The metachromasia requires water between the dye molecules to form the polymers and metachromasia does not usually survive dehydration and clearing.

Table 6.1 *Metachromasia and the spacing of acidic groups*

Material	Distance apart of acidic groups (μm)	Staining
Hyaluronic acid	1.03	Blue Orthochromatic
Pectic acid	0.5	Blue/purple Weakly metachromatic
Mast cell granules	<0.4	Red Strongly metachromatic

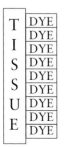 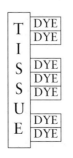 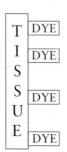

Figure 6.11 *Metachromasia. The tissue on the left would be metachromatic as the dyes have formed a polymeric form; the middle tissue would be weakly metachromatic as the polymeric forms are only a few molecules in size; the right hand tissue would be orthochromatic as the dye molecules are quite widely separated*

Examples of important dyes and their uses in histology stains

Nuclear stains

Nuclear stains are very important in histology as the structure of the nucleus is often altered in disease. It is also easier to recognize tissue structure when only the nuclei are stained than when other structures are stained but the nucleus is not stained. Nuclear stains are therefore important not only for looking at nuclear structure but also as counterstains for many other staining techniques since it is easier to recognize the location of the material in the tissue if a nuclear stain is used. For simple nuclear structure a blue haematoxylin stain is ideal. But for counterstaining it may not be the best option since a counterstain should have a totally different colour to the main technique so that it does not confuse identification. The blue/purple colours of haematoxylin often overlap with the colour of the main technique, so other nuclear counterstains are needed.

Haematoxylin

Haematoxylin is a natural product extracted from the heartwood of the tree *Haematoxylon campechianum* which was named after the Campeche state in Mexico where it was originally found. It is now cultivated in the West Indies. The logwood of the tree is first extracted with hot water and then the dye is purified by precipitation with urea. The dry powder is usually quite pure (about 95%) but it is not actually a dye. Haematoxylin is soluble in both water and alcohol but dissolves faster in alcohol, so stock solutions are often made by first dissolving the powder in alcohol and then diluting the alcoholic solution.

The formula of haematoxylin is shown below and one can see that there is no obvious chromophore and a solution of haematoxylin is not highly coloured.

Haematoxylin itself is not a dye and for staining the haematoxylin must first be oxidized to haematein. Haematein has two less hydrogen atoms and the rearrangement of bonds introduces the quininoid ring structure and hence colour as can be seen from the formula below.

Haematein is less soluble in water and alcohol than haematoxylin but is soluble in ethylene glycol and glycerol. Haematein is only a weak acid dye, imparting a yellowish colour to the tissues, but if it is combined with a suitable mordant haematein becomes probably the most widely used nuclear dye.

Strictly speaking the solutions called haematoxylin solutions are incorrectly named and should really be haematein solutions and haematoxylin-stained sections called haematein-stained slides but long usage means that the name haematoxylin will continue to be used.

Haematein itself can be further oxidized to oxyhaematein which is a weak acid dye but has no mordant dye capability.

Most working solutions do not completely oxidize the haematoxylin and the unoxidized part gradually oxidizes to haematein at the same time as some of the haematein oxidizes to oxyhaematein. This replenishes the working solution and greatly lengthens the life of the reagent. However, eventually all solutions will lose their strength and become useless. Oxidation is slower in acid conditions so many solutions are deliberately kept acidic. During the natural oxidation many haematoxylin solutions produce precipitates that must be removed by filtration before using the solution.

The oxidation of the haematoxylin to haematein can be done by atmospheric oxygen; a process called ripening. This is a slow process and can take months, especially in cold and dark conditions, so the ripening is slower in the cold, dark winter months than in the bright, warm summer sunshine. This ripening is considered to give a longer shelf-life but it is inconvenient if supplies run out since it may take months to prepare a new batch.

Oxidation can also be done immediately using oxidizing agents such as sodium iodate (200 mg per gram of haematoxylin), potassium permanganate (177 mg per gram of haematoxylin) or mercuric oxide (500 mg per gram of haematoxylin), though using smaller amounts than these traditional quantities will prolong the shelf-life as explained before. The oxidation with mercuric chloride needs heat (boiling) and can be hazardous if insufficient space is left to allow for the frothing that occurs on addition of the oxidizer to the boiling hot solution. Iodate and permanganate oxidation will occur at room temperature and do not cause the same frothing.

Mordants for haematoxylin

Haematoxylin is a very versatile stain and can be used to demonstrate many different tissue components in a highly selective way.

Brazilin, extracted from trees of the Caesalpina genus is very similar to haematoxylin (only one OH different) and can be oxidized to Brazilein. It can be used in the same way as haematoxylin but has never become as popular in histology. It is from this dye that the country of Brazil took its name.

BRAZILIN

BRAZILEIN

The type of mordant used alters the specificity and colour of the stain.

Aluminium salts: haemalum. These are the commonest haematoxylin solutions and there are many different formulae but they all have similar results. Typical formulations include Harris's, Mayer's, Ehrlich's and Gill's haematoxylins. The mordant is usually either aluminium potassium sulphate (potash alum) or aluminium ammonium sulphate (ammonium alum). Because of their use of alum salts as mordants these staining solutions are referred to as **haemalum** solutions. In acid solutions these alum dye lakes are quite soluble and have a strong red colour. In alkaline conditions the dye lakes are less soluble and have a strong blue colour. The dyeing bath is usually acidified and once staining is complete the section is rinsed in an alkaline solution to convert it to its blue form. This process is called **blueing** and makes the dye less soluble and more resistant to washing out. In hard water areas the tap water is alkaline and simply rinsing in tap water will 'blue' the section. If the water is soft then an alkaline solution can be prepared, e.g. lithium carbonate or tap water substitutes. The haemalums are used regressively with a controlled differentiation in acid alcohol (1% HCl in 70% alcohol) followed by reblueing in water.

Ferric salts: iron haematoxylin. The ferric salts used are either ferric chloride or ferric ammonium sulphate (iron alum). The resulting stain is blacker and more intense, and it will resist acidic counterstains such as van Gieson's better than haemalum solutions. The ferric salts are oxidizing agents and will accelerate the oxidation of the haematoxylin to haematein and this may result in over oxidation and loss of staining. The mordant is therefore either used separately (Heidenhain's) or the mordant and haematoxylin mixed just before use (e.g. Weigert's). Differentiation is often carried out using excess mordant and requires microscopic control. There is no need to 'blue' the sections in an alkaline solution since the mordant produces an intense black regardless of the pH. The use of iron haematoxylins has declined following the introduction of the celestin blue–haemalum sequence which also resists acid decoloration.

Other mordants which can be used to selectively stain certain tissue components are shown in Table 6.2.

Carmine and carminic acid

Carmine is a natural dye extracted from the red pigment cochineal that is used in cooking. Cochineal itself is extracted from the bodies of Coccus insects. Carmine is a complex of aluminium and carminic acid rather than just the dye molecule. Commercial carmine powder is quite variable in its composition and besides

Table 6.2 *Other mordants for haematoxylin*

Tissue element demonstrated	Mordant
Nuclei	Al or Fe
Myelin	Cr or Cu
Elastic fibres	Fe
Collagen	Mo
Neuroglia	W
Axis cylinders	Pb
Mucin	Al
Fibrin	W
Mitochondria	Fe
Heavy metals (Pb, Cu) and Ca	None (the metal in the tissues acts as the mordant and binds the dye)

the dye–aluminium complex also contains protein, calcium and other ions. Carminic acid is a glycoside with a glucose derivative joined to an anthraquinone structure.

Carminic acid is the pure dye and it is only slightly soluble in water but dissolves much better in solutions of an aluminium salt, when it forms the carmine complex. Solutions of the complex are not stable and significant deterioration occurs after only a few weeks of storage. For precise staining it is better if the carmine solution is prepared from purified carminic acid. Solutions prepared from impure commercial carmine powder are unreliable with some batches giving superb results and others being virtually useless.

For many years carmine was a major stain with its main advantage being its permanence when compared to other dyes. The problem with many other methods was that when they were mounted in Canada balsam the acidity of the mountant caused significant fading in just a few months. Carmine-stained sections are stable in acids and thus did not fade in this way and carmine was therefore very widely used. At the height of its popularity carmine was used for many different techniques and a great many methods were devised using it.

The unreliability of the dye supply and the rising cost of the natural product have led to it becoming much less popular. The loss of popularity has occurred at the same time as laboratories have switched to the use of modern synthetic mounting media that cause

In the preparation of the Romanowsky dyes methylene blue was used as 'polychrome methylene blue'. Polychroming involved heating a solution of the dye with a weak alkali (or sometimes performing other ill-defined procedures). The polychroming produces a range of dyes from the original methylene blue of which azure B is probably the most important. Modern Romanowsky stains generally use mixtures of pure dyes rather than the empirical polychromed methylene blue.

One of the methods used to produce polychromed methylene blue was to allow fungi to grow in a solution of it. The metabolic actions then converted some of the dye to other compounds. The relationship between dyes and micro-organisms can be quite interesting. Many dyes will certainly grow micro-organisms and this changes their staining character. Other dyes have been used as antibacterial agents and the selectivity of dyes led many people to believe that dyes might prove to be the 'magic bullets' that would kill selected bacteria and save humanity from infection.

much less fading of other dyes so there is less need for a stable nuclear stain.

A good carmine stain is easy for inexperienced workers to use since overstaining is difficult. Any excess dye can easily be removed with 1% HCl. The most popular stains were those for the carmalum techniques (e.g. Mayer, Grenacher) and acetocarmine.

Neutral red and safranine

These are popular red nuclear stains mainly used as counterstains to blue staining methods such as Perls method for iron. Both dyes are easily soluble in water and alcohol.

Neutral red can also be used as a vital stain when used at a very dilute (10^{-5}) concentration. Neutral red can also act as an indicator, changing colour at pH 6.8–7.0 (turns yellowish in alkali). Neutral red stains nuclei red and cytoplasm a pale yellow.

Methylene blue

This is a very widely used simple blue stain that does not require a mordant. It gives a quick and simple nuclear counterstain for red primary stains. It is readily soluble in water and alcohol. It can also be used as a vital stain provided a pharmacopoeia grade is used and it is also sensitive to reduction and oxidation (the reduced form is colourless).

It was a major component of Romanowsky stains used in the staining of blood smears and bone marrow specimens.

Methyl green

This blue/green nuclear stain is a useful nuclear counterstain and is also an important part of many techniques to differentiate between DNA and RNA in tissues. It is often contaminated with methyl violet but this can be removed by washing with chloroform.

Cytoplasmic stains

Cytoplasmic stains are often used as counterstains but can also be important to identify tissue components. Most techniques are also used to distinguish connective tissue fibres and other protein materials. The cytoplasmic stains should produce several different shades of colour so that the tissues can be easily distinguished. Most of the stains are acidic (anionic) dyes but can be used in mixtures to improve the contrast between different components.

Eosin

This is not a single dye but a variety of related dyes. All are derived from fluorescein which is a useful fluorescent dye widely used to label antibodies but which is useless for ordinary light microscopy.

Sodium fluorescein

By substituting halogens or nitro groups for some hydrogens a variety of shades of red can be produced from yellowish to bluish, e.g. eosin Y (yellowish) changes to eosin B (bluish) if the bromine groups on positions $2'$ and $7'$ are changed to nitro groups.

The dyes are also fluorescent but are solely used as red dyes. The sodium salts of the dyes are all freely soluble in water and fairly soluble in alcohol but will precipitate as eosinic acid if the pH is very low. Adding dilute acids to the staining will, however, improve eosin staining but may overdifferentiate the nuclear stain.

Eosin is a very good cytoplasmic stain as it gives several shades to the tissues. The range of shades can be extended even further if more than one dye is used in the solution. Some workers claim that up to seven different shades can be distinguished though I have always found it difficult to distinguish more than about four shades.

Eosin solutions keep reasonably well unless they are contaminated by fungi, when they will develop significant growths. This growth can be inhibited by adding a small amount of thymol to the solution and this acidic material also enhances the staining.

Ethyl eosin is an ester rather than the more usual sodium salt and is only slightly soluble in water. It is used when eosin staining is needed from alcoholic solution. It must be differentiated in alcohol. Eosin is also an important component of Romanowsky stains which are all eosinates of azure dyes. Its pre-eminent role in staining is shown by the fact that many structures are referred to as eosinophilic when they will stain equally well with other acid dyes.

Eosin gives a good red cytoplasmic counterstain but if other colours are required then other dyes must be used.

Methyl blue and aniline blue

These are widely used blue anionic dyes with similar staining properties. Both are water soluble but insoluble in alcohol. They are often confused as both are also known as soluble blue and water blue. Both are quite large dye structures and are frequently used to stain connective tissue fibres.

Fast green FCF and light green SF

These are green anionic dyes similar to the blue dyes above and are frequently used as counterstains to red dyes. Fast green FCF is less prone to fading than the light green SF.

Orange G, picric acid (trinitrophenol), metanil yellow and martius yellow

These are very pale-coloured dyes, ideal for faint background staining or in conjunction with other acid dyes. Orange G is soluble in water but less so in alcohol and is a major component of the Papanicolaou stain for cervical cytology.

Picric acid is also a fixative. It is soluble in water to a little over 1%, more soluble in alcohol and is a valuable stain in multiple acid dye techniques because of its small size. It is explosive when dry and care must be taken not to let any drying occur; this is especially important in the neck of bottles where the friction of opening can be enough to detonate any dried deposits.

Connective tissue methods

Connective tissues consist mainly of collagen fibres, elastic fibres, glycosaminoglycans and cells. The main way of distinguishing the fibres and cells is by using a combination of acid dyes to stain different structures in differing colours. There is still uncertainty about the exact mechanisms of these techniques (see, for example, Kiernan, 1990) but they seem to depend on differences in dye size and differing permeabilities of tissues.

Trichrome stains

The dyes used in trichromes differ in molecular size, e.g. picric acid (FW 229), acid fuchsin (FW 578) and methyl blue (FW 800) can be used as a trichrome mixture. The differing molecular weights and sizes affects their diffusion rate and their ability to permeate into small spaces in the tissues. The larger dyes will also be able to form more van der Waals bonds, so if two acid dyes are competing for binding to tissues the larger dye will generally tend to displace the smaller dye. Also the smaller dyes tend to be paler colours (yellowish) whilst the larger dyes are dense colours. Both of these effects combine so that smaller, paler dyes are overwhelmed by larger, denser dyes when they compete directly.

Tissue permeability is related to the amount of protein that is present and the amount of water between the proteins. Loose collagenous (areolar) tissue has many minute fluid spaces and is very permeable whilst red blood cells are packed full of haemoglobin and are much denser. Most other cells, including muscle, lie between these two.

The concept behind differential acid dyeing techniques is that only the small dye will penetrate into the dense red cells. The red blood cells should then stain with the smallest dye. In the less dense collagenous tissues the large and small dyes will be in competition. The larger dye will dominate and the collagen will appear to be stained only with the largest dye.

Van Gieson's stain

This stain uses two acid dyes each of which if used alone would stain all cytoplasm and connective tissues. By combining them in a single solution the tissue differences can be exploited. The open texture of the collagen allows free and rapid access to both dyes and stains red. Muscle and red cells, which restrict access of larger dyes, stain yellow. In van Gieson's stain both dyes are mixed into a single solution along with hydrochloric acid to give a pH of 1–2.

Permeability and dye size considerations would suggest that the small dye will rapidly penetrate both the dense red blood cells and the looser connective tissues. The larger fuchsin molecules will penetrate into the connective tissues quite readily but will penetrate the denser red blood cells only slowly. Where both dyes are present the fuchsin will displace or mask the paler picric acid with the result that the connective tissues will stain red, but in the red blood cells the picric acid will not be displaced or masked and the red cells will stain yellow.

Trichrome techniques

These take the differential staining a stage further and use three different dye sizes to selectively stain three tissue densities. The red blood cells are the densest tissue and stain with the smallest dye, the intermediate cytoplasm and muscle cells are stained red by the intermediate-sized dye and the collagenous tissues stain with the largest dye. In each case it is only the largest dye of the competing dyes that does the staining.

Heteropolyacids aid trichrome staining

Trichromes differ from van Gieson's stain in that an extra reagent is used in the form of one of the heteropolyacids. The hetero-polyacids are either phosphomolybdic (sometimes called molybdo-phosphoric) acid or phosphotungstic (tungstophosphoric) acid. One theory of their action is that these large ions act in the same way as dyes and clear the background by acting as 'colourless dyes' and displacing the intermediate molecular weight dye. These heteropolyacids improve the staining but whether they simply act as colourless dyes or have a more active role in some form of mordanting is still unresolved. Trichromes also differ in that the three dyes are usually used separately as a sequence of dyes rather than in a single mixed reagent as is the case with the van Gieson technique.

Trichromes can to some extent be 'tuned' to differentiate between tissue fibres by selecting dyes of appropriate sizes and by controlling the size of tissue spaces. Alcoholic solutions seem to affect penetration by allowing dyes to permeate more freely, possibly by increasing the tissue spaces. This makes the molecules act as if they were a slightly smaller size.

Molecular size and permeability: not the full story

Although the explanation given here accounts nicely for much of the staining with multiple acid dyes (trichrome and van Gieson) there are anomalies and the exact mechanisms are still very much undecided. In particular if the dyes are used alone they will quite readily stain all the tissues. The fuchsin dye in the van Gieson stain will stain red blood cells and this shows that it is able to penetrate these structures.

There is the possibility that the timing is crucial and that by using a limited time the red dye would not have long enough to penetrate into the cells. Even on theoretical grounds this seems unlikely; a red blood cell is less than 8 µm across at its widest and less than 3 µm thick. For diffusion across such small distances to take more than 2 min (which is a typical staining time for van Gieson's technique) would suggest a **very** dense material. If van Gieson staining is extended to 30 min or more there is no major difference in the result.

Similar anomalies can also be seen when different combinations of dyes are used. It is always the smallest dye that stains the red blood cells and the largest that stains the collagen. But the same dye can fulfil both roles in different situations. If acid fuchsin is used in combination with other dyes then the acid fuchsin will stain erythrocytes if the other dye is larger but will stain collagen and not erythrocytes if the other dye is smaller. The situation is more complex than the simple dye size and permeability would suggest, yet the concept does seem to hold in most practical applications and several very good trichrome methods have been produced on the basis of this theory.

Dyes and quality control

As mentioned earlier most dyes are not produced for histologists but for textile dyers. The important property for textiles is a reliable final colour and not chemical purity. Dye manufacturers therefore adjust their products to give consistent dyeing of fabrics rather than histological reliability. This means that dyes, unlike most biochemical reagents, are often impure materials and may contain significant amounts of other materials such as salts, dextrans and even other dyes. The actual content of the named dye rarely exceeds 95% and may be as little as 25% of the total weight. Different batches of dye will differ in their dye and contaminant content which makes quality control in the histological laboratory difficult.

The non-dye constituents are often very important and may often grossly affect the staining. To try to combat this problem some

Dyes have always been impure so it became important to have a good source of dyes. The dyestuffs are quite expensive to manufacture so it was not unknown for dyes to be 'cut' with less expensive materials to make them more profitable. Some older samples of dye certainly seemed to have an insoluble residue left after preparing the staining solution. One manufacturer (Grübler), however, became famous for the quality of his stains and if you read the old textbooks you would find his dyes being recommended time after time in techniques as being the best available. Nobody thought his dyes were purer, just better. It was said that 'not only does Herr Grübler have the best dyes he also has the best impurities'. Grübler dyes lost their leading role following the Second World War when the importing of dyes from Germany became impossible and laboratories had to find other sources.

laboratory suppliers offer **Certified Dyes** that have been tested biologically for their stated uses. Such dyes are more expensive but should match their stated uses reliably.

Also it is worth repeating that some dyes have many names and it should always be made clear which dye is needed by using CI numbers, otherwise the dye may be completely different. When a staining method suddenly stops staining as you expect, it is worth checking that you have not just got a different batch of dye to the usual one.

Checking dyes in a histology laboratory

Quality control of dyes within the laboratory is difficult since many of the techniques used in quality control require complex equipment to analyse the dye samples (e.g. infrared spectroscopy, HPLC) but some simple tests can usually be performed.

- **Chromatography.** This will detect coloured contaminants of dyes and can be a sensitive way of comparing two dye batches. Simple paper chromatography using filter-paper is often enough to pick out impure dye samples.
- **Measurement of absorption** (including a full spectrum if a suitable spectrophotometer is available) can be used to determine the amount of dye in a sample and may also show contaminants.
- **Testing with standard dyeing techniques** can determine if the dye is suitable or needs altered staining times/conditions. Some dye batches may be suitable for one stain but not others, for example fuchsin samples may be all right for use in ZN staining for mycobacterium but not for preparing Schiff's reagent.

Once a dye is made up into a solution it may not be permanently stable. Dyes can alter due to oxidation by the air, bleaching by light, contamination by micro-organisms growing in the solution or chemical reactions between constituents of the dye solutions. So even when the dry dye is acceptable the dye solutions made from it may be unsuitable if it is not fresh or is stored inappropriately.

Reagent bottles should be clearly labelled with the date of preparation and renewed at regular intervals or sooner if the staining seems to be suffering. If light accelerates the deterioration then storage of the reagent in brown bottles to prevent light reaching the dye may help, but the dark glass also masks any contamination and precipitation so you still need to be careful. Most techniques which have reagents that need special storage (e.g. refrigeration) will usually give appropriate details.

Silver impregnation

Metallic impregnation is an alternative way to increase the contrast in tissues. The commonest metal to use in light microscopy is silver which produces a dense black, fine deposit of silver and silver oxide where the silver ions have been reduced. Silver impregnation is also called silver staining but the mechanism is quite different to the effects of dyes and the structures are actually plated with the silver rather than the silver being reversibly bound to the section.

Advantages

Silver impregnation has a number of advantages compared to dyeing techniques and has a number of very common applications. The main advantages of silver techniques are:

- They are stable and do not fade. The end product is a metallic silver which, if properly fixed and washed, is effectively permanent. The silver deposit in black and white photographs is similar to the material produced by silver impregnation and photographs from 150 years ago are still in excellent condition. Dyed sections rarely last more than 10 years without some signs of fading.
- The silver deposit is densely black which provides good contrast and is excellent for taking photographs.
- Silver techniques are very sensitive methods and will detect many materials that are difficult to demonstrate by dyeing. These materials include reticulin fibres that are difficult to observe with haematoxylin and eosin but can be well demonstrated with silver impregnation. Metal impregnation methods are more common in neurological methods, e.g. for observing axons, motor end-plates and astroglia.
- Slender objects are thickened because they become silver plated. This can be useful for fine fibres such as reticulin or for slender bacteria such as spirochetes.

Disadvantages

Silver techniques also suffer from certain disadvantages:

- They can be unreliable and capricious. The techniques will sometimes work well and other times they will not work at all. This can extend to different workers. There sometimes seems to be one person in the laboratory who can get a technique to work perfectly but everyone else struggles even when using the same reagents. Staining times can vary tremendously from one day to the next when a fresh batch of silver solution is prepared.
- The silver solutions are often very alkaline solutions. Strong alkaline solutions have a tendency to strip sections off the glass slides so extra care and adhesives are needed.
- Silver techniques are so sensitive that they can sometimes give non-specific background deposits ('dirty preparations').
- They have a tendency to stain everything they come into contact

with (hands, laboratory coats, benches, glassware etc.). Silver is very difficult to remove without using dangerous reagents so clothing is often permanently stained. The silver solutions are easy to wash out if they are caught early enough but since they appear just like water it is not always obvious that there has been a spillage. Once the silver has been reduced the safest way to remove silver deposits is by using an iodine solution that converts the silver to silver iodide and the silver iodide is then soluble in sodium thiosulphate solutions.

- Some silver solutions have a tendency to become explosive if stored for more than 24 h.
- Silver is expensive.
- Silver salts cannot be discarded into the mains drains as silver is a heavy metal poison.

Why use silver and how it is used

Silver is not the only metal that can be used for impregnations but is the most useful as it is easily reduced, and any reduced silver acts as a catalyst for the reduction of more silver. This autocatalytic activity makes silver useful in many fields other than histology. The use of silver is widespread in photography and the chemistry of photography and silver impregnation are very closely related.

The silver solutions are reduced during the impregnation so silver techniques are primarily methods for reducing materials. There are three different ways to produce the silver deposits. These are the argentaffin reaction, the argyrophil reaction and ion exchange reactions.

The argentaffin reaction

In the argentaffin reaction the tissue contains reducing groups that are sufficiently strong and present in sufficient quantity to give a visible silver deposit without the need to add any reducing agents. This is found particularly in the reducing pigments and is strongest with the enterochromaffin pigment that derives its alternative name (argentaffin pigment) from the reaction. The strong reaction in this case is due to phenolic components (5-HT). The reaction only needs the addition of the silver solution, such as in the Masson–Fontana technique, but tends to be very slow and may take up to 24 h to give a deposit.

The Argyrophil reaction

Many tissue groups are able to absorb silver, possibly by ionic mechanisms as for dyeing. The silver is mainly absorbed as silver ions but small amounts are reduced to silver atoms. These silver atoms are deposited at the site of the reduction. This initial

Figure 6.12 *Silver deposition and reduction in the argyrophil reaction*

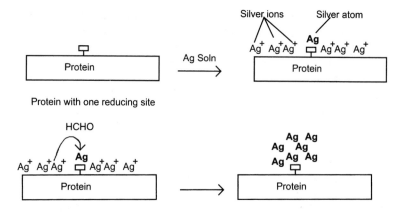

reduction reaction with silver only deposits submicroscopic atoms of silver at particularly reactive sites. Probably only a few, perhaps as few as two, atoms of silver are deposited in this initial stage and these are too small to be visible even with high power microscopy. The silver atoms then act as catalytic sites where more silver can be deposited by the reducing action of a developer (Figure 6.12), e.g. formaldehyde or hydroquinone (quinol). In this case the main reduction is done by the developer and the tissue simply provides places where there are silver atoms to catalyse the reduction. Without any silver atoms to act as catalysts the reducing agent reacts too slowly to give a visible deposit. This type of reaction, where an external developer is added, is called an argyrophilic reaction.

Ion exchange reactions

Ion exchange can also deposit silver and this is used to detect mineralization of bone using the von Kossa technique. The section is treated with silver solution (silver nitrate) and the phosphates and carbonates in mineralized bone form insoluble silver salts. The silver salts are then blackened by UV light or hydroquinone solutions. Although often said to demonstrate calcification of bone the method really detects carbonates and phosphates.

$$CaCO_3 + 2\,AgNO_3 \longrightarrow Ag_2CO_3 + Ca\,(NO_3)_2$$

$$Ag_2CO_3\ (\text{UV treated}) \longrightarrow Ag_2O + CO_2$$

$$\text{Black}$$

Silver solutions

Ammoniacal silver solutions are used as they are easily reduced. Silver solutions always need careful preparation and some diammine silver solutions can become explosive if kept for more than 24 h. If they are being used in a glass container then a simple safety precaution is to wrap them up with adhesive tape (Sellotape) then, if an explosion occurs, the glass fragments are held by the sticky tape. It is important to always use distilled water in any silver method as tap water will react with the silver salt.

Several silver solutions can be used in silver techniques but they are not directly interchangeable as they differ in their sensitivity to reduction.

Silver nitrate

This is the commonest form of silver salt used in the preparation of silver solutions. Simple silver nitrate solutions are sometimes used, e.g. von Kossa, or they can be part of sensitizer solutions, e.g. Beilschowsky's method for nerve fibres, but for most techniques a more easily reduced form of silver salt is needed.

Silver diammine

Silver diammine solutions are prepared by precipitating the silver with a hydroxide solution and then redissolving in a minimum amount of ammonium hydroxide. These solutions are very alkaline and this makes sections more liable to detach during staining so an adhesive is often advisable. The final solution can be explosive if it is stored for more than 24 h. These solutions have the advantage of being very sensitive.

$$2\,Ag^+ + 2\,OH^- \longrightarrow Ag_2O + H_2O \qquad \text{Precipitation of silver oxide}$$

$$Ag_2O + 4\,NH_3 + H_2O \longrightarrow 2[Ag(NH_3)_2]^+ + 2\,OH^- \text{ Dissolving to form diammine silver}$$

Silver carbonate

Silver carbonate solutions are prepared by precipitating the silver using either a lithium or sodium carbonate solution. The precipitate is filtered and washed. This removal of the precipitating salt is different to the previous example with silver diammine where the hydroxide is left in the solution. The precipitate is then dissolved using strong ammonia as for the previous diammine solution. Silver carbonate solutions are claimed to be even more sensitive than the diammine solutions.

Hexamine silver solutions

These use hexamine (methenamine, hexamethylene tetramine). When mixed with silver nitrate this produces a white precipitate that immediately redissolves without the need to titrate with strong ammonia.

Background deposits

Silver techniques often produce a non-specific deposit due to contaminants. Very small deposits can often be reduced by **toning**. This involves using 'gold chloride' (sodium chloroaurate).

$$3\,Ag + (AuCl_4)^- \longrightarrow Au + 3\,AgCl + Cl^-$$

Thus three silver atoms are replaced by one gold atom. For very small deposits this will result in a great reduction in size (reduced background) but the large deposits of the impregnated tissue will hardly be affected. Gold toning also alters the colour from an intense black to a warmer brown/black colour.

Following completion of the technique the sections are usually treated with 'hypo' (sodium thiosulphate, previously called hyposulphate). This is photographic fixer that dissolves excess silver ions and prevents them later depositing as background. It is probably not necessary in histological preparations since all the silver is usually completely reduced so there is little risk of further reduction, but it is always done 'just in case'.

Silver techniques

Reticulin can be demonstrated using silver impregnation and, for such demonstrations, the following is a fairly typical technique. First the reticulin is oxidized to give aldehyde groups:

Then the silver solution oxidizes the aldehydes to acids and in the process is itself reduced to silver atoms which precipitate at the site of reduction:

Aldehydes are one of the commoner reducing groups in tissues and silver solutions can often be used to detect the presence of aldehydes.

Silver techniques vary quite widely in their conditions

There are many variations on silver techniques that seem to give good results. It is largely a matter of preference which technique

works best in a particular laboratory. There are probably differences between the laboratories that are not particularly mentioned
or even controlled which make one method more suitable for one
laboratory than another. These variations include tissue fixation
and processing, water quality (both tap and distilled or de-ionized
water), ambient temperature and ambient light.

The actual concentrations of silver involved vary quite markedly
from 1 g per 100 ml (Foot) to 10 g per 100 ml (Laidlaw). Times and
temperatures also vary from 30 s (Gordon and Sweet) to 60 min
(Perdrau), and temperatures range from room temperature of 20 to
70°C (Lillie).

This wide variation might suggest that the technique was quite
insensitive to conditions and the method would work reliably
regardless of any slight technical errors. This is not the case.
Silver techniques are more difficult to get exactly right than most
staining methods and require care, patience and experience to get
an even impregnation and lack of non-specific background. The
wide variation is a reflection of this, since many people have tried,
and largely failed, to get an automatic and reliable technique.

General treatment of sections during staining

Paraffin wax sections after drying to achieve adhesion are still not
ready to be stained since they are totally impregnated with wax
which forms a waterproof coating and prevents dye access to the
proteins.

Section rehydration

For staining the wax must be removed and the section rehydrated.
This is conveniently done using stainless steel racks which hold a
number of slides and flat staining dishes. The dry, labelled slides are
placed in the rack and the wax is removed. Xylene is still the most
commonly used reagent for this process. Xylene is less commonly
used for processing tissues because of its tendency to cause
shrinkage and hardening. There is no problem with shrinkage at
this stage since the tissues are now firmly attached to a rigid slide,
and hardening is no longer a difficulty as there is no further
sectioning to be done. Removal of the wax needs to be complete
since if any wax remains it will result in uneven staining. Treatment
with xylene for 5 min is usually sufficient.

The tissues can then be transferred through a series of graded
alcohols (typically 100%, 95%, 70%) and finally into distilled
water. They do not need prolonged times in any of these baths
since penetration is very rapid through the thin sections; 30 s with
gentle agitation will usually be enough.

This process of returning a paraffin section to water is usually
called either dewaxing or 'taking the section to water', or is

If the section is frozen then the phrase 'take the section to water' can be ignored since the section is already in water. Often students do not think and try to process the tissue as if it was a paraffin section and this can totally ruin the section. For that reason I personally prefer the phrase **'take the section to water'** to **'dewaxing'** as it is less prescriptive and suggests that the histologist needs to get the section into water from the medium the section is currently embedded in.

Sections are best dewaxed immediately before being stained. Once rehydrated they will slowly deteriorate especially if kept in water. Deterioration is not rapid and sections can be kept in water, alcohol or xylene for quite long periods but they do gradually lose adhesion. This is similar to the 'soaking' of pans with dried-on food residues. Since soaking will remove dried-on food it is hardly surprising that it will also remove dried-on sections.

It is also a bad practice to allow sections to dry out at any stage in the staining as this can introduce minute air bubbles into the protein mesh that is the cellular structure. These air bubbles may remain and are not removed when the tissue is again placed into reagent and end up in the final preparation. There are occasional instances when sections need to be dried but these are the exception.

occasionally known by the somewhat grander phrase of **deceration**. One of these phrases will be found at the beginning of most staining schedules and must always be done when paraffin sections are used. Once fully rehydrated the sections can be stained in aqueous reagents until they are ready to be mounted.

Automated staining

As well as automating processing it is also possible to automate staining. The same general principles apply to both situations. Automation frees staff from a routine task which is relatively straightforward and allows them to do more demanding tasks. The use of an absolutely regular procedure ensures that there is little variation in results so that direct comparisons are valid from one batch of stained sections to the next. This accuracy and reproducibility are crucial in some applications such as diagnostic and exfoliative cytology (Chapter 12) where the colour of the cytoplasm is an important diagnostic feature.

The disadvantage is that there is less flexibility. All the sections will be given the same treatment regardless of their needs. It is also only feasible for techniques that are done in large numbers. The machines are fine for doing hundreds of haematoxylin and eosin stains but it is not reasonable to use a machine for stains where the technique is only required for two or three slides each day. It also does not lend itself to situations where different results are needed. For example when photographing at low magnifications an over-stained section will give better results than the usual staining intensity. An ordinary stain will give insufficient contrast for the film's recording capabilities but a more intense stain will give stronger differences between the tissues.

Automatic staining machines are also less flexible in producing single stains even when they are already programmed for that stain. So producing a single slide may hold up some types of machine and these machines must go through the full cycle before another section can even begin since the steps are uneven. These machines are inefficient for staining single sections. An alternative strategy is to have all the steps the same length (say 1 min) and then sections can be added at any time and will follow the same path. The difficulty here is that if a longer time is needed then several baths of the same reagent are needed. These machines often cannot cope with large numbers of sections in a short space of time.

Automated staining is very useful for absolute regularity with large numbers of sections needing the same treatment at the same time. They have found a significant role in two main areas:

- Haematoxylin and eosin staining in histology, Papanicolaou staining in cytology and blood film staining in haematology. This is because the sheer numbers needing staining make it worthwhile.

- In immunohistochemistry, nucleic acid hybridization and similar techniques. Here the actual numbers are smaller but the need for absolute consistency is greater so there has been a move to more automation.

The use of automatic coverslipping machines is often linked to automated staining. The process of mounting sections is very mundane so automation is possible. There is less requirement for variety in mounting so, provided they are working well, these machines are a useful addition to the laboratory.

Section mounting

Mounting of sections under a coverslip is essential to get the best and clearest view of the specimen. You only need to compare an unmounted wet section at the end of staining with a properly mounted section to see the difference. The microscope manufacturers usually assume that the specimen will be mounted in a medium with a high refractive index and covered with a thin glass coverslip and actually calculate all their optical corrections on that basis. The difference can be seen in Figure 6.13 where the optical paths through a wet section and a mounted section are compared. The unmounted section has twice as many refracting surfaces and the opaque tissue will transmit much less light.

The coverslip should have a thickness of 0.17 mm (No. 1 coverslip) for the best results since this is the thickness used by microscope manufacturers in their calculations when designing lenses. Thicker coverslips such as No. 2 will marginally interfere with the clarity and very thick coverslips may even prevent the oil immersion lens being used, as they can have a greater thickness than the normal working distance of the oil immersion lens.

Mounting media

The mounting medium used under the coverslip should have a high refractive index (RI). Most tissues have an RI of between 1.5 and 1.55 so a mounting medium with a refractive index in this range will give maximum clarity. There is no single mounting medium that will be suitable for all specimens and all stains. There are two

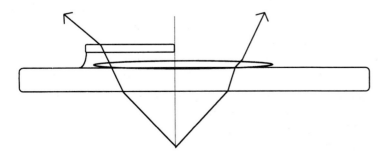

Figure 6.13 *The effect of a coverslip on sections. On the left a section mounted in a high refractive index medium has only two refractions whilst a section in water has up to four refracting surfaces*

major types of mounting media used and the difference is in the solvent. The commonest types are the resinous mounting media that are based on hydrophobic organic solvents, usually xylene, and which need the section to be dehydrated and cleared before mounting. Water-based mounting media will accept tissues straight from distilled water and are used when a xylene-based medium would not be appropriate, e.g. if the dye or histochemical reaction product is soluble in xylene.

The properties that need to be considered in a mounting medium are:

- **Refractive index.** If the RI is much lower than 1.5 then tissues will not be completely transparent and diffraction will occur. This is usually a disadvantage as it reduces clarity but it can sometimes be an advantage as it will give some contrast to even unstained tissues.

- **Clarity under normal conditions of use.** Some media can become opaque as they dry out and are not suitable for long-term preservation.

- **Effects on the stain itself.** Some mounting media will cause fading. This is most common with acidic mounting materials that will cause significant fading especially in the light. Some media may also act as solvents for the dyes and, as a consequence, the dye diffuses or leaches out into the mountant. This will gradually obscure the tissues.

- **Low fluorescence or non-fluorescent.** This is only critical for fluorescence microscopy but it is generally a useful characteristic for a general mounting medium since it eliminates the need to use a special mountant when fluorescence is being used.

- **Setting.** The ability of a mountant to dry or set quickly and hold the coverslip in place is very useful. Many aqueous-based media fail to harden sufficiently and the coverslip will need ringing to preserve the section.

Resinous mounting media

Canada balsam. This was the original resinous mounting medium used in histology. Canada balsam is derived from the *Abies balsamea* fir tree and is available as a dried, brittle, yellow solid. It will melt at high temperature and is soluble in xylene, and about 60 g in 100 ml of xylene gives a good working mountant, though it takes a few days to completely dissolve. The yellow colour of the mountant hardly seems to matter when viewed through the microscope. It dries somewhat slowly but holds the coverslip well. Prolonged storage will result in total evaporation of the xylene and it may result in some crystallization so specimens mounted in Canada balsam are usually ringed to prevent evaporation. The mountant is usually significantly acid and will cause fading especially of basic dyes. It is relatively expensive and is mainly of historical importance rather than being a common mountant.

DPX. This is a synthetic polystyrene resin that is dissolved in xylene and has some plasticizer added. The initials come from the term Distrene 80 (a commercial polystyrene) Plasticiser (e.g. dibutyl phthalate) Xylene. It is a water-white, clear solution and is one of the more popular mountants in use. It has very little tendency to fade dyes and hardens in about 24 h and does not need ringing.

Other synthetic media are available such as 'Permount' or 'Entellan' which are commercial brand names.

When a section comes to the end of normal staining and is to be mounted in a resinous mounting media it needs to be dehydrated and then cleared in xylene before being finally mounted. This is simply the reverse of the dewaxing but it is better not to use the same reagents as they gradually become contaminated with the other reagents, e.g. dewaxing will leave wax in the xylene which can interfere with the mounting medium.

Aqueous mounting media

There is no fully satisfactory aqueous medium and several different ones are used for different purposes. They differ in the way in which the RI of water (1.33) is raised sufficiently to give a clear image. Most are best considered as temporary mounts and need ringing to hold the coverslip in place and prevent drying out. Tissues do not need any treatment before mounting and can be mounted directly from water or buffer.

Glycerol. Glycerol is a trihydric alcohol with a high refractive index. It can be simply used alone or with the addition of a buffer to control the pH. It is a useful medium for fluorescent staining such as the immunofluorescent antibody techniques. The addition of *p*-phenylenediamine is said to retard the fading of fluorescence. It neither hardens nor dries out and is usually used as a very short-term mountant though it can be ringed if it is to be kept.

Glycerol jelly. This uses the addition of gelatine (up to 12% in some formulations) to allow the medium to set. The usual formulation has a lower RI (1.42) than most mounting media so the clarity is reduced and some unstained structures will be visible. It is solid at room temperature and needs to be melted in a water bath before use. It is very easy to get air bubbles trapped within this medium so it is convenient to melt it and get rid of air bubbles by warming it in a vacuum embedding oven. Glycerol jelly is quite a good growth medium for some bacteria and fungi so there is usually an antibacterial additive (e.g. phenol) but it will still not keep well. Sections may similarly grow organisms in storage so it is best thought of as a temporary mount.

Apathy's medium. This uses a gum (gum arabic or gum acacia) and sucrose to raise the RI. It has a refractive index of around 1.5 so it can give nicely transparent preparations. It has a tendency to crystallize in storage and although it does set by drying this is quite slow. It may again need the addition of an antibacterial agent to help preserve it.

Polyvinyl alcohol or polyvinylpyrollidone medium. These are synthetic and less liable to bacterial contamination than the organically based mountants though the addition of phenol is still advisable. They dissolve in water or buffer but need constant stirring. They solidify slowly by evaporation or they can be ringed. These are more permanent than the other water mounting media but are still not as good as a resinous medium.

Temporary mounts need ringing

Ringing is the term used for sealing the edges of a coverslip when the mounting medium does not set. Ringing was originally so called because the coverslips were round and so there was a ring of the sealant round the coverslip. Ringing was done on a turntable to give a nice neat finish. Originally it used a gold size followed by a black asphaltum varnish. This produced a very neat finish and some commercial suppliers of prepared slides still finish many of their preparations in a similar way since it looks good. Most laboratories have dropped this and ringing is now just a temporary expedient rather than an aesthetic requirement.

Good temporary ringing can be achieved in a number of ways. Ordinary nail varnish works quite well and comes in a bottle with its own brush which makes it convenient and simple. The only drawback is that it is dissolved in acetone which might affect some materials but I have never found it to be a problem. Many styrene-based cements can also be used and again are convenient since they come in tubes ready to squeeze out round the coverslip. The solvent is a theoretical problem but again I have not had problems. These can often be semipermanent and slides may be kept for several weeks. Paraffin wax can be used. A piece of warmed metal (such as the flat end of a broad spatula) is used to apply a layer of molten wax which immediately sets. Provided the slide is dry this is quick and easy but is easily broken and will not store well.

Slides should always be carefully labelled and stored horizontally until fully dry when they can be stored on their edge or end. Store stained slides away from light as the dyes will fade even in the best mountant.

Suggested further reading

Horobin, R.W. (1996). The theory of staining and its practical implications, in *Theory and Practice of Histological Techniques* (eds J.D. Bancroft and A. Stevens). Edinburgh: Churchill Livingstone.

Kiernan, J.A. (1990). *Histological and Histochemical Methods.* Oxford: Pergamon.

Self-assessment questions

1. What is the role of chromophores and auxochromes in dye structure?
2. How do basic and acidic dyes demonstrate the structure of tissues?
   Name one acidic and one basic dye.
3. How do pH and salt concentration alter dye binding?
4. A small amount of mordant allows staining and excess mordant removes the staining.
   Explain this oddity.
5. Why does haematoxylin mordanted with aluminium salts stain nuclei but other mordants cause haematoxylin to stain connective tissues or nerve fibres?
6. Toluidine blue will stain mast cell granules red.
   What is the name of this phenomenon?
   Why does the colour change occur?
7. Name one red and one blue nuclear stain.
   When would you use a red nuclear stain and when would you use a blue one?
8. Why do some haematoxylin solutions initially improve with keeping and then deteriorate?
9. Outline why permeability and dye size might explain trichrome staining with three acid dyes.
10. Distinguish between argentaffin and argyrophil silver impregnations.
11. Why is silver the best metal for metallic impregnation techniques?
12. Why might a lipid staining technique recommend mounting in glycerol jelly instead of DPX?
13. Why do most laboratories routinely use a resinous mounting medium?

Key Concepts and Facts

Staining
- Staining is used to give contrast between different components of tissue.
- Staining allows the tissue structure to be examined by visual microscopy.

Mechanism of Staining
- Staining involves bonding between tissues and dyes.
- Ionic bonding is the most important form of bonding in histological staining.
- Ionic staining distinguishes between basophilic and acidophilic tissue components.
- Hydrogen bonds and van der Waals forces are less important than ionic bonds but play a role in selectivity.
- Ionic staining requires that both tissues and dyes are ionized.
- Two or more dyes can be used in combination to give better contrast between materials.

Dye Structure
- Dyes are ionic, coloured, organic molecules.
- Chromophores give dyes their colour and auxochromes give dyes the ability to ionize.
- Dyes are usually given trivial names and can be impure and inconsistent in their properties.

Mordants and Metachromasia
- Mordants are metallic salts that help bind some dyes to tissues.
- Haematoxylin is the most important mordanted dye and is the most important nuclear dye.
- Metachromasia produces a different colour in the tissues to the colour of the dye solution.
- Mordanting involves polymerization of the dye in the tissues.

Silver Impregnation
- Silver impregnation uses silver salts to produce contrast in tissues.

- Silver methods are very sensitive and can be used to demonstrate many materials better than dyeing methods.

- Silver can react with tissues by an argentaffin, argyrophil or ion exchange mechanism.

General Treatment of Sections
- Paraffin wax sections must be dewaxed and rehydrated before staining ('taken to water').

- After staining sections are usually mounted in a transparent mounting medium and covered with a coverslip.

- Water mounting media allow mounting directly from aqueous solution and help to preserve some hydrophobic materials.

- Resinous mounting media are usually dissolved in xylene and sections must be dehydrated and cleared before they can be used.

- Mounting media not only protect the specimen but also make it translucent and easier to examine.

Chapter 7

Histochemistry: general considerations and the histochemistry of carbohydrates and lipids

Learning objectives

After studying this chapter you should confidently be able to:

Outline the problems associated with identifying and localizing chemicals in tissue sections.

Describe the periodic acid–Schiff (PAS) reaction and be able to outline the problems in interpreting the PAS reaction.

Describe how to identify and localize mucins in cells and tissues.

Describe a histological classification of mucins.

Describe how lipids can be demonstrated in tissues.

Histochemistry is a method of investigating tissue structure which, instead of using relatively crude dyeing of the tissues, uses reasonably specific chemical tests to identify and pin-point the location of chemicals within the tissues. In this regard histochemistry is a modified form of chemistry or biochemistry.

Histochemistry and biochemistry

Histochemistry may have a lot in common with biochemistry but it has certain extra problems since biochemists investigating tissues usually have some quite significant advantages over histochemists.

- Histochemistry must produce a coloured final result to make it visible under the microscope. Biochemists can certainly employ methods that produce coloured final reaction products but they can also quite happily employ methods that use materials only 'coloured' in the ultraviolet region - and such results are invisible to the human eye and useless for microscopy.

- Histochemistry must produce a material that is insoluble so that the position of the chemical reaction in the tissue can be accurately located. Slight solubility of the final material is a problem since it can allow the coloured material to move from its true site to a nearby location and give a false localization.

- Histochemistry must be highly sensitive as it must accurately detect the material present within a single cell and in some cases within a single organelle such as a mitochondrion. Biochemists can often use several kilograms of tissue to make a single preparation and concentrate the material they are investigating.

- Histochemistry must never allow the materials to be separated from their environment since pin-pointing their position in the tissues is the whole reason for using histochemistry. The biochemist can separate and purify the materials using a range of techniques such as chromatography, electrophoresis and dialysis. Indeed the very speed of the movement in such separation techniques is often the best method of identifying closely related materials.

Histochemistry is therefore often more difficult to achieve in practice and is often less certain in its identification than the equivalent biochemical detection. It is also much more difficult to get an accurate quantification (see the section on Microscopical measurement in Chapter 15). So it is best to think of biochemistry and histochemistry as techniques that supplement each other rather than being competing techniques; they give different information and when used together give a more complete picture of the chemistry of the cell than either could alone. Biochemistry can determine what materials are present in a tissue and in what quantities, whilst histochemistry can identify the position and distribution of the materials. Histochemistry also relies on the knowledge gained from biochemistry to enable satisfactory histochemical techniques to be developed.

Use of controls in histochemistry

Controls are important in histochemistry and should include a minimum of a **positive control** and a **negative control**. Without controls the methods are little more than demonstration techniques which though still useful cannot be considered as rigorous chemical testing.

Positive controls

The purpose of a positive control is to check that the technique is working satisfactorily. For this purpose you need a weakly reacting

If many different tissues are being examined together then the number of control sections can become tedious. In some cases it is possible to have a large number of control tissues yet only one control section. The method is to pack a large number of test tissues into one block. The tissues may be simply blocked-out separately in one mould or by cutting small rods of tissues they can be assembled into a single checker-board or composite block. For control purposes you only need a very small sample of tissue to see if the technique is working as expected, so as little as a square millimetre of tissue will suffice. A single checker-board may contain 64 separate tissue samples in a single section. This is an effective way to reduce the number of control slides without compromising the number of control tissues. The only disadvantage is the time and effort needed to make the composite blocks.

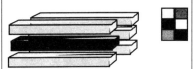

Rods of tissue are assembled into a solid block and when sectioned appear as a checker-board of tissues.

material. The reason for using a positive control is to ensure that any material in the test section will be detected. If a strongly reacting control is used then it is possible that the test is working for a strong reaction but is insensitive to a weak reaction. A strongly reacting control may also be included to give a good positive for comparison but it should be in addition to a weak control not a replacement. Where a material may have several forms that react differently (such a case would be amyloid which has a number of different types), then it may be necessary to control with more than one positive material. So for amyloid the controls may include both of the common AA and AL amyloid types (see Chapter 14) and perhaps even some of the less common types if they are likely to occur in one or more of the test sections.

Where a technique is being used quantitatively then the use of a range of controls is needed to cover the range of results expected and to act as a standard for the quantitation.

The positive control should be as close as possible to the material being looked for in the test section. For example, using the PAS technique it would be possible to check that the technique is working by using glycogen or a mucin or reticulin fibres or several other materials. If you are looking for glycoproteins in the pituitary then the control should be glycoprotein in the pituitary not glycogen in the liver. The use of a totally different material is not as good a control since the materials may react differently.

The positive controls should be carried out at the same time and in the same way as the test sections. It is not enough to control the technique once at the beginning of the day and then use the result for several different batches of tests run at different times. A single positive may be sufficient for a batch of sections which are tested at the same time provided the test sections are similar in type and in the reaction expected.

Negative controls

Negative controls are used to test the specificity of the reaction and ensure that there are no false positive results. The tissue should again be as close as possible to the test section in type and in expected reaction. In many cases it is often possible to use another slide of the test section as a control by destroying the reactivity (see Treated tissues below). It may be necessary to have a negative control for each section if there is some background colour that might be confused with the positive result. Only by comparing the negative and test sections can you be sure that the result is a genuine positive.

Control results

The controls should always be examined first. If the results are satisfactory then the test slides can be examined and reported.

If there is any sign of a positive result in the negative control then the method may not be specific and some factor other than the test material may be reacting. If the positive control is negative, or unexpectedly weakly reacting, then the method may not have been sufficiently sensitive or may have been performed wrongly. In both cases the tests will need to be repeated. The controls may need to be investigated first to ensure that the results can be relied on before repeating the tests again.

A simple rerun of the controls is a useful start, taking extra care to ensure that all the steps are carried out correctly. This will detect if the results were due to a simple error in technique. The rerun can be done using fresh reagents to ensure that it is not a reagent error and different control slides to ensure that it is not a control section error. If the rerun fails to give the expected results then the whole technique needs to be reassessed. Each step may need to be controlled separately to detect which step is going awry. This may result in a huge number of controls but is the only way to ensure reliable results.

Controls can be of various types

The source of controls is important and it is sometimes necessary to use different types of control tissues especially when investigating unexpected results.

Control tissues

Positive control. This involves having tissues which you know contain the material you are demonstrating. The material can be a sample from a previous test that came up positively. Most laboratories are constantly looking for good positive control materials to use in subsequent tests. The use of stock controls assumes that the material is stable enough to be kept. Some control materials do deteriorate during storage and may need regular replacement.

If the material cannot be stored or if there is no stock control available then it may be necessary to use fresh animal tissue. This would be the case for enzyme techniques where it may not be possible to store tissues since the enzymes do deteriorate quite quickly. It is then essential to use a tissue that you are certain contains the material.

Negative control. Here it is essential to choose a tissue that does not contain the material being demonstrated to check for non-specific reactions. Ideally the negative tissue should be from the same organ and the same species as the test sections.

Treated tissues

These are an excellent negative control since the actual tissue under test is treated to remove or destroy the staining ability of the material. This can be used not only to ensure that the method is specific but also when the method is known to be non-specific. For example, the PAS technique is useful but stains many different materials and is not specific for glycogen. It can be used to demonstrate glycogen specifically by using a control in which the glycogen is removed by enzyme digestion with amylase. Other PAS-positive materials such as mucins, glycoproteins and reticulin will be unaffected. So a material that stains in both the test and treated tissue control is not glycogen. Any staining which is positive in the test but missing from the amylase-treated tissue is glycogen. These controls are not so easy to examine and interpret as totally negative control sections but this type of destructive controlling is a vital method in many histochemical investigations.

The material can be destroyed in a number of ways:

- Enzyme digestion, e.g. amylase for glycogen, collagenase for collagen, ribonuclease for RNA.
- Extract with a solvent, e.g. chloroform/methanol will dissolve lipids.
- Specific inhibitor, e.g. oxaloacetic acid will specifically inhibit succinic dehydrogenase but not inhibit other enzymes.
- Heating to destroy enzyme activity, e.g. acid phosphatase by Gomori's lead phosphate technique. Any coloration will be non-specific binding of the lead salts.
- Blocking of reactive groups. This may involve reacting the group with reagent, e.g. acetylation of hydroxyl groups (use acetic anhydride in pyridine). The term is also loosely applied to complete removal of the group, e.g. deamination with nitrous acid.

Altered technique

It is possible to ensure that there is no non-specific reaction by simply omitting an essential step in the technique. For example, an easy negative control for an enzyme is to omit the substrate from the incubating solution. The absence of substrate means that the enzyme cannot catalyse its normal reaction so any positive result is non-specific. Similarly omitting the periodate oxidation in PAS acts as a good test for any preformed aldehydes.

These types of controls are very useful in investigating unexpected positive results. By omitting different steps in the procedure it is often possible to identify the source of the unexpected reaction. This control of individual steps is used in immunological and related techniques where there may be six or seven steps that could be the source of the false positive reaction.

> The blocking methods are also used to prevent background reactions by removing the reactive material before performing the test. So preformed aldehydes in tissues can be blocked by reduction with borohydride. This is useful, for example, after glutaraldehyde fixation when there are many free aldehydes from the glutaraldehyde. The use of any method using Schiff's reagent which detects aldehydes is therefore difficult unless these abnormal aldehydes from fixation are first blocked.
>
> The use of blocking is also employed in immunoperoxidase methods to destroy endogenous peroxidases (Chapter 10).

Histochemical investigations

Histochemical tests as simple staining methods

Many histochemical techniques are used in routine histology not so much for the chemical information they can provide as for the fact that they are often better at showing a particular object than simple dyes could ever be. Examples include the use of acetyl cholinesterase techniques to demonstrate motor end-plates, the PAS technique to show goblet cells, nucleic acid techniques to identify plasma cells and lipid techniques to show myelin degeneration. In these cases the histochemical controls are often omitted since the technique is not being used in its most critical way. This should not be taken to mean that the controls are never necessary, just that they can be omitted for simple demonstration methods but would still be needed for more rigorous histochemical testing.

Staining techniques in conjunction with histochemical investigations

It is also true that many staining techniques that are not strictly histochemical are often used in histochemical investigations where they may confirm the results of another test. Two or more non-specific tests may between them give results that are quite acceptable as histochemical identification even though individually they are not specific. Thus Alcian blue will stain many forms of mucin and aldehyde fuchsin will stain many materials including sulphated mucins, elastic fibres and some cell inclusions. If a material stains with Alcian blue and with aldehyde fuchsin (in separate sections, not in the same individual section) then it can be safely assumed that the material is a sulphated mucin. Individually the two techniques are not specific but their combined results are at the very least highly selective.

Whether to fix and how to fix

In all histochemistry, as indeed in all histological investigations, the early treatment of the tissue is vitally important. Improper treatment of the tissue, such as inappropriate fixation, will result in the material under investigation being altered, moved or even completely lost. Since histochemistry involves more precise chemical investigation it is very often done on unfixed tissue. This means that the tissues are unstable and must be used quickly. Once the histochemical reaction has occurred and the final insoluble product is formed then it is often possible to post-fix the tissues to make them more permanent.

Histochemistry is sometimes perceived as being difficult and obscure. This is not true. Histochemistry is not always difficult or complex. The Perls technique for iron is one of the most sensitive of the histochemical techniques. In this case ordinary paraffin wax sections will suffice since the material being identified is protein-linked and therefore retained in paraffin sections. The reagents are not complex or critical and I use the technique in first year degree practical classes. It works reliably for the students. They can observe the iron present within the spleen cells. Individual macrophages can be distinguished easily in their preparations.

Any technique that can be done first time every time by inexperienced workers and still detect the minute amounts of iron present inside a single macrophage can hardly be called difficult. Not all histochemistry is so easy but a surprising amount can be performed with little difficulty given reasonable care.

Materials for histochemical investigation

There are a number of reasonably specialized subdisciplines within histochemistry each of which has its own problems and solutions. These include the histochemical identification of:

- carbohydrates;
- lipids;
- nucleic acids;
- proteins;
- enzymes;
- pigments;
- minerals.

Carbohydrates

The carbohydrates found in tissues are mainly sugars and their derivatives. Simple sugars such as glucose and fructose are extremely difficult to preserve in tissue sections as they are very soluble in water. Distinguishing between simple sugars by chemical tests is quite difficult and glucose is also almost ubiquitous in cells and tissues. The identification of free monosaccharides is rarely attempted in tissues since the sugars are likely to have been lost or moved from their original site and any positive reactions are likely to be the glucose that is known to be everywhere.

Sugars can, however, be bound to a number of other materials to give a range of sugar-containing materials which are of interest to histochemists. The presence of any sugar can usually be identified by the **periodic acid–Schiff (PAS) technique**. This is the single most important technique in carbohydrate identification since it identifies most neutral sugar and sialic acid-containing materials. It does not, however, identify the type of sugar that is present but simply indicates that a saccharide is present.

Periodic acid–Schiff (PAS) reaction

The PAS reaction involves a two-step chemical reaction in which there is first an oxidation in periodic acid to generate aldehyde groups from the carbohydrate and this is then followed by a sensitive reagent for aldehydes (Schiff's reagent) to finally stain the site of the sugars.

Periodate oxidation

The oxidation acts on the glycol (hydroxyls on adjacent carbons) part of the sugar and produces two aldehydes and at the same time splits the bond between the two carbons:

$$
\begin{array}{c}
\text{H–C–OH} \\
| \\
\text{H–C–OH} \\
|
\end{array}
+ IO_4^- \longrightarrow
\begin{array}{c}
\text{H–C=O} \\
\\
\text{H–C=O} \\
|
\end{array}
+ IO_3^- + H_2O
$$

Reaction with Schiff's reagent

The aldehydes then react with Schiff's reagent to produce a product that is a strong purple colour. The reaction can also occur with some derivatives of sugars and glycols, e.g. amino and alkylamino sugars. Most materials that contain sugars, such as a glycoprotein, will be PAS-positive. Strongly sulphated mucins in connective tissue and hyaluronic acid are negative with the standard PAS technique despite containing large numbers of sugar groups but other mucins are PAS-positive.

Agents for the oxidation

Periodic acid (HIO_4) is the most commonly used oxidant and is made up as a 0.5% or 1% aqueous solution (0.044 M) and oxidation is for 5–10 min at room temperature. A longer oxidation may be needed for some materials to become Schiff reactive (e.g. sulphated mucopolysaccharides). Adding extra steps to the technique may also increase the range of materials demonstrated (e.g. borohydride treatment). Alcoholic periodic acid can be used instead of the aqueous solution if there is the possibility of the material dissolving in water (e.g. Hotchkiss in 1948 recommended alcoholic periodate oxidation for glycogen).

Other oxidants can be used to give the same reaction but most will also cause further oxidation of the aldehydes to acids with consequent loss of staining. This further oxidation does not happen with periodic acid and it is this that makes periodic acid the most popular reagent. Other oxidants that can be used include chromic acid, potassium permanganate, lead tetra-acetate and sodium bismuthate. These oxidants need more precise timing to obtain maximal staining and it is this critical timing which makes them much less popular, but they are occasionally included in other staining methods, for example chromic acid oxidation is used in the Gridley technique for fungi.

Schiff's reagent

Schiff's reagent is a sensitive reagent for detecting aldehydes and stains them a pink/purple colour. It is quite specific for aldehydes. Even the related ketones do not react with the PAS method. The Shiff's reagent consists of a solution of basic fuchsin (pararosani-line) which has been decolorized with sulphurous acid. The sulphurous acid adds an extra sulphurous group to the central carbon of the dye. This disrupts the chromophore group with consequent loss of colour.

Pararosaniline with
the quininoid chromophore
as the bottom ring

Schiff's reagent
has no quininoid ring
and is colourless

On reacting with the tissue it seems likely that the alkylsulphonic derivative of the dye is formed. This entails a rearrangement of the sulphonic group and restores the chromophoric group, but this is not simple restoration of the original dye colour since the product is a significantly different colour to the original dye.

> The PAS reaction is such a useful indicator that it is one of the few stains where a negative result is often given and many cellular components will be described in the books as PAS-negative. The negative result means no sugars are present so it acts as a method of distinguishing glycoprotein hormones from simple proteins, e.g. in the pituitary.
>
> This use of the negative result is quite unusual and means that it is used in situations where you expect no reaction. In such cases controls need to be more stringent than normal since a negative result is expected and poor technique will give a negative result.
>
> Other techniques that have this distinction include Sudan staining and the Perls method. It is also the case with the Gram bacterial stain where Gram-negative indicates a great deal about the bacterium.

The quininoid ring chromophore is restored
when the Schiff's reagent interacts with an aldehyde

To prepare Schiff's reagent therefore requires a solution of basic fuchsin or pararosaniline. The fuchsin needs to be specifically for the preparation of Schiff's reagent as not all 'basic fuchsins' are suitable. The starting concentration of the dye solutions usually contain 0.5–1% of dye. At concentrations lower than 0.5% the Schiff's reagent does not seem sufficiently sensitive to detect all the aldehydes but 0.5% seems adequate to show all the reactions and is the recommended concentration for quantitative work.

Varieties of Schiff's reagent

The sulphurous acid needed to decolorize the dye can be produced in various ways:

- Sulphite or metabisulphite and HCl at 50°C (de Thomasi). This is one of the most popular recipes.

- Metabisulphite and HCl at room temperature with prolonged shaking (Lillie). This 'cold Schiff' is more acidic than the previous recipe.

- Thionyl chloride (Barger and Lamarter).

- Bubbling sulphur dioxide through the solution (Itikawa and Oguru).

- Sodium dithionite (Alexander).

Sensitivity and shelf-life

Although they all produce effective reagents there are differences in their sensitivity and shelf-life. The amount of sulphurous acid seems to be the main difference affecting the Schiff's reagent. If there is an excess of sulphurous acid then it gives better keeping qualities but may reduce sensitivity of the Schiff's reagent. Schiff's reagent should be stored at 0–4°C when it may keep for months.

After the sulphurous decolorization the Schiff's reagent is often a yellowish colour and this can be removed by treating the solution with activated charcoal. A slight yellowish tinge does not seem to matter and the Schiff's will still work fine, but if a pink colour is produced it indicates degradation of the reagent and it should be discarded. Because of the hassle involved in preparing Schiff's reagent many laboratories now prefer to buy the reagent from a commercial supplier.

Washing out

In the original techniques the Schiff's reagent was washed out of the tissues using sulphurous reagents as a rinsing solution. For most routine purposes the use of sulphurous acid rinses after the Schiff's reagent has largely been dropped in favour of simply washing in running water for several minutes, but sulphurous rinses may be needed for critical applications. The water wash generally increases the intensity of the colour as any excess sulphurous acid is removed.

Alternative reagents

A PAS-stained section can be counterstained in many ways but the use of a nuclear stain such as haematoxylin is usually sufficient. The traditional Schiff's reagent prepared from fuchsin or para-rosaniline can be replaced by reagents prepared with other dyes such as thionin. Instead of Schiff's reagent the aldehydes can be detected with a silver reagent, usually methenamine (hexamine) silver. This is called PA-silver but is less popular.

Interpreting the results of a PAS reaction

Many materials are PAS-positive and if badly carried out the PAS technique can also give false positive results – so controlling and interpreting the results are very important before relying on the PAS technique as a method of identifying a material.

False positive reactions

The first type of false PAS reaction is given by an improper Schiff's reagent. If all the dye has not been decolorized or if the Schiff's reagent is old, then the section may develop a pink colour independent of any aldehyde. This should not happen if the Schiff's is correctly prepared, is reasonably fresh and has been stored correctly. The Schiff's reagent should always be examined for signs of deterioration before it is used but deterioration of the reagent is always a possible explanation if results seem unusual.

The second type of false reaction occurs when there are pre-formed aldehydes within the tissues before the periodic acid oxidation. Such aldehydes will react with the Schiff's reagent and give the same colour as if it was a PAS-positive substance. Preformed aldehydes can come from the use of an aldehyde fixative. Formaldehyde fixation is not normally a problem since the formaldehyde is effectively washed out of the tissues during processing, but other aldehydes, particularly glutaraldehyde, can cause difficulties.

Preformed aldehydes also occur naturally in small amounts in tissues and, particularly after mercuric chloride fixation, they can appear as the so-called **plasmal** reaction. The plasmal reaction is mainly due to lipids ('plasmalogens') and so this is more likely in frozen sections but can sometimes occur in paraffin sections. Blocking of fixative-derived or preformed aldehydes is possible, e.g. using sodium borohydride, but is not a common procedure.

To ensure that non-specific reactions are not occurring a second section can be carried through the technique but omitting the periodic acid oxidation. Any material or component stained in both sections is not PAS-positive but indicates something else, usually a preformed aldehyde.

False negative reactions

The cause may be a reagent that is not working effectively or inadequate treatment with one or more reagents. A positive control section, where you are sure the material is present, should be stained alongside the test section to ensure that the technique is working. The control should be a weak rather than a strong positive and should be as close in type and material to the test section as is possible.

A negative result when a positive reaction was expected may also be due to a poor technique; staining a slide upside-down is an example. The test should be repeated ensuring that no errors occur.

The materials may have been lost due to processing or delayed fixation. If this is the case the only way to correct it is to get a new specimen.

PAS-positive materials

Some of the more commonly met materials that can be PAS-positive are shown below. This is not a comprehensive list but indicates the range of materials that need to be considered when a positive reaction is found.

Amyloid
Basement membranes
Cartilage
Cellulose
Cerebroside lipids
Chitin
Epithelial mucins
Fungi (chitin)

Glycogen
Hyaline membrane of neonatal lung
Lipochrome pigments
Pituitary basophil granules
Starch
Thyroid colloid
Zymogen granules in pancreas

If the PAS is being used for a specific confirmation then the identity of the material will probably be obvious. The problem of identification can arise if there is an unexpected positive reaction or if the identification of a material needs to be confirmed beyond doubt.

There is no simple procedure to be certain of the identity of a PAS-positive material. Several techniques can be applied:

- Simple appearance can often be useful. Some PAS-positive materials can simply be recognized by their shape (morphology), e.g. fungal hyphae are sufficiently distinctive for their morphological appearance to be enough for a positive identification.

- Stain a second section with another technique that selectively stains the material which you believe is the source of the PAS reaction. Starch can be identified by treating it with iodine when it will develop a distinctive blue colour. Even if the other technique is not itself specific the combination of PAS reactivity and staining with a second technique may be unique, e.g. lipochrome pigments also stain with ZN technique and Sudan black. So anything that stains positive with all three methods can be identified as lipofuscin.

- Dissolving or destroying the material chemically, e.g. dissolving glycolipids in hydrophobic solvents shows that they are soluble in organic solvents and this is a strong indication of their lipid nature. This requires two sections to be stained together. One section is pretreated with a lipid solvent and after the extraction both sections are stained with the PAS technique. Materials which stain in both sections are not glycolipids since they are insoluble in the lipid solvent. Glycolipids will show positively in the section that was not extracted but will not stain in the treated section.

- Enzyme digestion. Really this is the same as above but enzymes are such precise reagents that it can be a positive identification and is therefore worthy of separate consideration. This is useful for glycogen. Diastase (amylase) specifically digests glycogen and starch. Since starch is not a normal constituent of animal tissues this makes it highly selective and starch can be eliminated by iodine staining. Predigesting one section with amylase and comparing with an undigested section (both of which have been stained by PAS) allows identification of the glycogen. It also of course eliminates glycogen as a possible material when both sections are positive.

Specific carbohydrates found in tissues

Polysaccharides: glycogen and starch

Glycogen is the major form of carbohydrate found in human tissues and acts as the main energy store in many cells such as muscle and liver. Glycogen is one of the commonest materials giving a PAS-positive reaction in tissues. Glycogen is a polymeric form of glucose (the glucose is linked mainly α-1,4 in straight chains but there are some α-1,6 links which give some branched chains). It is related to starch which has the same general chemical composition but is generally found as bigger polymeric molecules. Since only one type of unit (glucose) makes up these materials they are termed homoglycans. Two forms can be identified by electron microscopy:

- α-glycogen which forms distinctive rosettes of β-particles;
- β-glycogen in which the individual components of the rosettes are free as individual 20–40 nm particles.

Glycogen is found in many cells with large amounts in liver and muscle cells.

Glycogen relocation within the cell during fixation

Glycogen illustrates an important characteristic of histochemistry, namely the role of fixation in the successful demonstration of a tissue material. The preservation of glycogen is important. If it is improperly fixed glycogen can be lost completely or its location within the tissue can be disturbed. The routine fixation with formaldehyde is not ideal since some of the glycogen is lost so the amount left in the section is diminished. The glycogen is also relocated by 'streaming' in the cytoplasm and becomes polarized within the cell. In streaming the glycogen is effectively washed to the far side of the cell by the fixative where it then becomes fixed. Using an alcohol-based fixative retains more glycogen and

Glycogen is quite variable in tissues as it is continuously used as an energy source by cells. The amount of glucose can alter quite markedly depending on diet and activity. Long-distance runners attempt to manipulate their glycogen stores by eating a high protein and low carbohydrate diet until shortly before a race. The lack of dietary carbohydrate depletes their liver and muscle cells of glycogen since protein cannot be easily converted into carbohydrate by the cell's metabolism. Then, for a few hours before the race, they will eat a high carbohydrate diet that causes the cells to actively store as much glycogen as possible.

This carbohydrate loading means that they can have maximum glycogen stores for the race. Glycogen is a much more available energy store so that muscles will be that little bit more efficient than if they were running on lipids, the next available source of energy.

diminishes the streaming artefact (Gendre's fluid is recommended as giving better results). However, the best preservation is achieved by avoiding fixation altogether and using freeze-drying to prepare the tissue.

Starch is usually a contaminant

The presence of starch in animal tissues usually means contamination of the specimen, the commonest source being the glove powder used in many rubber gloves to make them easier to put on. The starch can be distinguished from glycogen by staining with iodine (starch is blue, glycogen is brown); also starch is usually in the form of grains that show Maltese-cross birefringence with a polarizing microscope.

Cellulose

Cellulose is another homoglycan of glucose but linked β-1,4. It is usually found in plant materials but this can include cotton wool, gauze, filter-paper and clothing so cellulose fibres are amongst the commonest contaminants of tissues. Cellulose fibres are usually easy to recognize: they are PAS-positive, birefringent, insoluble in all common reagents and resistant to enzyme digestion by amylase.

Chitin

Chitin is a homoglycan of *N*-acetylglucosamine linked β-1,4. It is found in the exoskeleton of invertebrates. It is of only minor importance in mammalian histochemistry where it only occurs as either a contaminant or as part of a complete invertebrate parasite.

Many PAS-positive substances are protein–sugar combinations

Many of the most important compounds containing sugars are mixtures of protein and sugars. These can be many and varied in form, structure and function. They are studied by many different disciplines and this has led to a variety of nomenclatures that don't always agree with each other. One simple distinction is between glycoproteins and proteoglycans. The major distinction here is between the dominant chemical in the combination:

- **Glycoproteins** are proteins that have some sugar added as a post-translational modification but are predominantly protein. They are widespread as membrane proteins where the sugars act as stoppers to prevent the proteins slipping back through the membrane. The sugars always occur on the outside of the cell and form the **glycocalyx** (the carbohydrate cell coat) where they act as antigens and cell recognition structures. They also occur as

Starch was originally used to replace the mineral talc as a glove powder. Glove powder is needed with latex gloves to allow them to slip on to the hands easily. Talc is a magnesium silicate and remained in the body and could cause problems including 'talc granulomas'. Starch was used to perform the same task as it is more easily degraded in the body. Starch has now been found to have lesser but still significant problems and can delay wound healing. The Medical Devices Agency in the UK recommended that the use of powdered gloves should be discontinued. Gloves made of plastic that is not as sticky as rubber latex is now common in surgical practice. Laboratory gloves may still use glove powder and in other countries the use of glove powder is still common.

serum proteins such as immunoglobulins, structural proteins such as collagen and as secretions both exocrine and endocrine. Their histochemical properties are mainly determined by the protein but they do give a positive PAS reaction.

- **Proteoglycans** are mainly carbohydrate in nature with a small protein core surrounded by large polysaccharide chains. It is this group that has confusing nomenclature and are often known in histology by the imprecise terms of mucins or mucopolysaccharides. The histological classification of mucins that will be followed here is that of Cook (1974).

Mucins

Mucins are a group of substances that have certain physical, chemical and staining characteristics in common. They all contain large amounts of sugars attached to a small amount of protein and they all stain PAS-positive. Many mucins also react with the dye Alcian blue at acidic pH and many show metachromasia and this forms the basis of the histological classification.

Histological classification of mucins

The histological classification of mucins is based on staining properties and two major groups of mucins can be identified (neutral and acid mucins).

Neutral mucins

Neutral mucins are PAS-positive but are Alcian blue-negative and display no metachromasia with thiazine dyes such as toluidine blue.

Acid mucins

Acid mucins are PAS-positive and also stain with Alcian blue and demonstrate some degree of metachromasia. Acid mucins can be further subdivided on their staining behaviour with regard to pH due to the type and number of the ionizable acidic groups.

Strongly sulphated acid mucins. These stain with Alcian blue and are metachromatic even at very low pH (less than pH 1). They are mostly connective tissue mucins, e.g. cartilage, chondroitin sulphates, keratan sulphates.

Weakly sulphated mucins. These stain with Alcian blue and are metachromatic only when the pH is greater than 1, e.g. epithelial mucins in colonic goblet cells.

Weakly acidic (carboxylated) mucins. These stain with Alcian blue and are metachromatic only when the pH is greater than 2.5, e.g. epithelial mucins of salivary gland and the connective tissue hyaluronic acid. They can be further subdivided by the type of acid group (either uronic acid or sialic acid) and these can be identified by enzyme digestion with hyaluronidase or sialidase followed by Alcian blue staining.

Identification of mucins

Identification of mucins is most conveniently done by using several staining techniques. The routine stains such as PAS and Alcian blue give information that is useful but they can be even more useful if more than one technique is applied to the same section in a sequence so that the techniques interfere with each other and effectively compete for the carbohydrate.

PAS results

This is positive for all groups of mucins. However, if the mucin is first stained with another technique (e.g. Alcian blue) the dye will prevent or block the PAS reaction and the mucin will not then stain PAS-positive.

Alcian blue result

This is a cationic dye with an unusual structure (it is a copper phthalocyanine dye) and if the pH is kept acidic it will only stain acid mucins. It does not stain nuclei, probably due to the size and shape of the dye and the conformation of the DNA. Although other cationic dyes can be used to stain mucins it is this lack of nuclear reactivity combined with a strong colour which resists fading which has made Alcian blue so popular in staining mucins. By varying the pH or salt concentration, Alcian blue can identify the different types of mucin.

Aldehyde fuchsin result

This stains substances containing sulphur groups a strong purple colour. It will stain sulphated mucins very strongly. It will also stain many other tissue components purple (e.g. elastic fibres) even though they are not mucins. So only components that stain with Alcian blue and which will also stain with aldehyde fuchsin can be classified as sulphated mucins. By staining with aldehyde fuchsin first it is possible to inhibit or mask Alcian blue staining. The mechanism for the affinity of aldehyde fuchsin for sulphated mucins is not known and the stain should be regarded as an empirical test (i.e. no rational reason) but it does seem to work reliably.

Mucins are normally very useful materials but if the body loses the ability to destroy the mucins then they will accumulate and cause severe disruption. This happens in a number of uncommon diseases called the mucopolysaccharidoses. These are inherited gene defects in which the affected individuals accumulate mucinous substances inside and between cells. The accumulations occur because of an enzyme defect in the lysosomes. The severity of the disease and the type of accumulated material depends upon which enzymes are defective or missing.

Affected babies often appear normal at birth and may develop normally at first. It is often only when the child seems to develop frequent infections that the disease is diagnosed. The effects are progressive but vary widely in their severity.

Patients often develop coarse facial features (hence the term 'gargoylism' for these diseases). Thick skin and unusual hair growth also disfigure these patients. Skeletal involvement often causes distortion of the body. Corneal abnormalities are not uncommon and can lead to impaired vision. Internal organs may enlarge, e.g. the liver (hepatomegaly) and spleen (splenomegaly). There will be mental retardation in severe cases. Their overall growth is usually stunted and their life expectancy is usually short.

There are several variants of the disease of which the best known are Hunter's disease and Hurler's disease.

Critical electrolyte concentration

This technique uses differing concentrations of magnesium chloride (or different pH levels) to inhibit Alcian blue staining in mucins. The dyes are made up in the appropriate concentration of the salt as shown below and then used to stain sections.

$MgCl_2$:	pH:	Type of mucin:
<0.06 M	>2.5	All acid mucins Alcian blue-positive
0.2–0.3 M	1–2	All sulphated mucins Alcian blue-positive
>0.5 M	<1	Only strongly sulphated acid mucins Alcian blue-positive

If a group of sections is treated with the range of concentrations then it follows that if a mucin is stained in all the conditions then it is a strongly sulphated mucin. If a mucin stains in the first two solutions but not in the highest concentration then it cannot be a strongly sulphated mucin and must be a weakly sulphated mucin. If it only stains Alcian blue-positive in the weakest concentration of salt then the mucin must be a carboxylated mucin.

Combining the techniques

By combining these techniques it is possible to identify the major groups of mucins.

Alcian blue–PAS. The Alcian blue blocks the PAS reaction in acid mucins and so distinguishes between neutral and acid mucins. Acid mucins stain blue and neutral mucins stain purple from the PAS.

Aldehyde fuchsin–Alcian blue. The aldehyde fuchsin stains the sulphated mucins dark purple and the carboxylated mucins take up the Alcian blue.

The finer distinctions are made by using enzymes to differentiate between the carboxylated mucins and the critical electrolyte technique to distinguish between the strongly sulphated and weakly sulphated acid mucins (see Scheme overleaf). This scheme looks easier to do than it is in practice. The colours can sometimes be vague and inconclusive, some mucins react poorly in practice and there are conflicting results in some cases. Nonetheless the scheme is useful for identifying mucins.

Fats and lipids

Lipids are usually defined by their solubility in fatty solvents and their insolubility in water. Solubility is referred to by the terms:

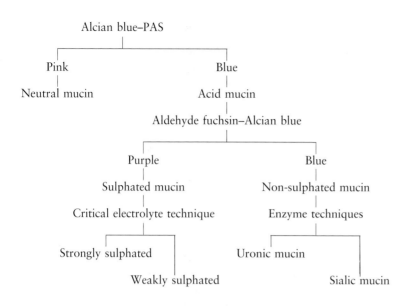

Scheme: *To identify mucins staining two sections with Alcian blue–PAS and aldehyde fuchsin–Alcian blue allows identification of the major mucin types*

- **hydrophobic** which refers to materials that are insoluble in water but soluble in organic solvents;
- **hydrophilic** which refers to materials which are soluble in water but not soluble in organic solvents;
- **amphipathic** which refers to materials that have parts of the molecule which are hydrophobic and parts which are hydrophilic.

All lipids are therefore at least partly hydrophobic but are otherwise often quite varied and they frequently have very little in common except their solubility. For example, the differences in structure, distribution and function between a steroid hormone such as testosterone and the adipose fat found in the subcutaneous tissues are much greater than the similarities in their solubility. Nevertheless in histological terms the solubility has been of crucial importance. The identification and location of lipids is generally less well understood and less frequently investigated histologically because the traditional wax sectioning techniques remove all the lipids. It is almost a truism to say that lipids are materials that cannot be investigated in paraffin wax sections. Because lipids cannot be investigated in paraffin wax sections most histologists have historically chosen to investigate other things.

Types of fats and lipids

The classification and structure of lipids have been confused and different methods of grouping the various types have been used. Metabolically there are two types of lipid and these are the **steroids** which have a complex ring structure as the hydrophobic part of the molecule and those lipids in which the hydrophobic part of the

Even though fats are soluble in the solvents used for clearing they can still cause problems in the cutting of wax blocks. Lipids will act as a waterproofing and will prevent the complete dehydration of blocks that are rich in fats. The fat itself will be gradually dissolved by the clearing agent and the block will then be left incompletely dehydrated. The water content may be very small but unless the clearing agent is water-tolerant and can complete the dehydration the final block will have some water trapped within the tissues. During storage this water can evaporate and the tissue shrinks, leaving a depressed block.

If there is much fat then it may not be completely dissolved by the clearing agent. The final block will be improperly impregnated and will not section easily if at all.

molecule is an aliphatic fatty acid. In many biochemical textbooks these two materials are dealt with quite separately since the metabolic pathways dealing with steroids are completely different to those dealing with the fatty acids. Histology textbooks more commonly use a classification that is based on whether the lipid is conjugated or not. In many of the demonstration techniques used in histology the critical difference is often whether the lipid is a hydrophobic lipid or an amphipathic lipid.

Conjugated and unconjugated lipids

The lists below show the categories of lipids which are conjugated (esters or amides) and unconjugated.

Conjugated lipids:
1. Neutral fats
2. Waxes   Hydrophobic lipids
3. Cholesterol esters
4. Phosphoglycerides

   Phosphatidyl choline
   Phosphatidyl ethanolamines
   Phosphatidyl serine
   Ether phosphatides   Phospholipids   Hydrophilic lipids
   Phosphatidyl inositol
   Diphosphatidyl glycerols

5. Sphingomyelins
6. Ceramides
7. Glycolipids

Unconjugated lipids:
1. Fatty acids
2. Steroids   Hydrophobic lipids

   Cholesterol
   Steroid hormones

Section preparation for lipids

The first thing that must be considered in investigating lipids is how can they be preserved and sectioned?

Fixation is difficult for lipids

Most of the fixatives used in histology are protein fixatives and do not fix lipids; at best they leave them unaffected (e.g. formaldehyde) at worst they may even destroy them (e.g. alcohol). Only two fixatives have any significant fixative action on lipids and neither is commonly used. The first is osmium tetroxide which adds on to double bonds in tissues including those in unsaturated lipids.

$$H-C \atop \|\ + OsO_4\ \longrightarrow \atop H-C \qquad {H-C-O \atop H-C-O}{>}Os{<}{O \atop O}$$

This fixes the lipid but also blackens it. This makes osmium-fixed lipid unsuitable for most histochemistry. Osmium tetroxide is, however, very important in electron microscopy since the fixation and blackening preserves and stains membranes that are a vital part of the ultrastructure of cells.

The second fixative that can preserve lipids is potassium dichromate which can preserve some phospholipids though it has little effect on triglycerides or steroids. This has been used in histochemistry in the Marchi technique and the Baker technique for phospholipids but otherwise the prolonged dichromate fixation needed to fix the phospholipids is not common.

The majority of lipid histochemistry is therefore done on unfixed lipid because, even if the sections have been fixed to preserve the protein, the fixatives usually have no effect on the lipid. The sections are usually cut frozen and this means that the best fixative is formaldehyde which allows good frozen sections and does not alter lipids. The addition of 10% calcium chloride is believed to help preserve phospholipids but fixation should be kept short (< 2 days) to prevent the formation of soaps with free fatty acids. Fixation is often delayed until after sectioning (or even after staining) when fixation times can be considerably reduced.

Sections are virtually always prepared by a frozen section technique with cryostat sections generally being preferred and fixation being done after cutting.

Neutral lipid staining

Simple neutral lipids can be localized very easily using **lysochrome** methods that rely on the hydrophobic nature of the lipid. Lysochrome staining involves using a dye that is very soluble in lipids but relatively insoluble in aqueous solvents. If the dye is made up in an aqueous solvent then when it is applied to the tissues the hydrophobic dye will become concentrated in the tissue lipids even when it is only at a low concentration in the watery phase. Such a solution of a hydrophobic dye will rapidly colour the lipid by a simple solution mechanism whilst leaving the hydrophilic proteins and nucleic acids uncoloured since it is much more soluble in the hydrophobic lipid than in the aqueous solvent (Figure 7.1).

The first techniques used in this way relied on Sudan dyes (Sudan I, II, III, IV) so this type of reaction is often called **sudanophilia**. Only Sudan III and IV were ever popular in histology and these have now been replaced by an even more highly coloured and hydrophobic dye, oil red O. In either case the hydrophobic dye must be dissolved in high concentration in an aqueous solvent in which it

Figure 7.1 *Process for neutral lipid staining*

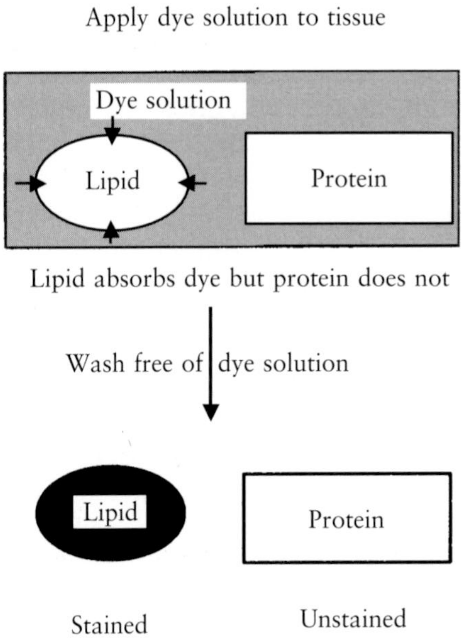

Apply dye solution to tissue

Lipid absorbs dye but protein does not

Wash free of dye solution

Stained   Unstained

The staining of lipid is one method of determining if a person died instantaneously in an accident even if they are not examined until many hours or days later. In an accident in which bones are broken the fatty material in the bone marrow will be released into the bloodstream. The fatty material does not dissolve but remains as solid fat embolisms. The embolisms are carried round in the bloodstream until they reach a capillary, where they lodge. The first capillary bed the droplets encounter is usually in the lung. So in a fatal accident if a fresh section of lung is taken and stained by a lysochromy technique then the finding of lipid droplets from the marrow shows that the heart went on beating after the bones were broken so the person did not die immediately.

is not very soluble. This contradiction means that it is not usually a simple solution.

One of the earliest reliable techniques was that of Herxheimer who used acetone and alcohol. This has significant solvent ability for the dye but unfortunately it will also dissolve some lipids. It gives excellent demonstration of major fat deposits such as adipose tissue but may dissolve very small droplets of lipid such as might be found inside non-adipose cells.

Lillie and Ashburne introduced isopropanol as a solvent. The stock solution of the dye is a saturated solution in 100% isopropanol but for use the stock solution is diluted immediately before being used to give a final concentration of 60% isopropanol. This weaker alcoholic solution has much less solvent action on the lipid but in diluting the stock a supersaturated solution is produced which gives a high concentration of dye. The supersaturated solution is unstable and must be used immediately.

Chiffelle and Putt used propylene glycol and Gomori used triethyl phosphate, both of which are claimed not to dissolve lipid though they will dissolve the dyes.

Most laboratories use one of these three techniques depending mainly on personal preference.

Since all the solvents use the dye at close to saturation it is important to filter the dye solutions to remove any precipitate and to prevent evaporation during staining which would cause deposits to occur. Removal of excess dye solution is usually done with the same solvent that was used for the dye and this is then followed by washing in water. This rinse in solvent helps to prevent any precipitation of the dye and keeps the background clear. The dyes used are red and are usually counterstained with haematoxylin.

Temperature alters lysochrome dye solubility

Staining at room temperature will demonstrate neutral lipids but not most phospholipid, cholesterol or their derivatives which are crystalline at room temperature. These can be rendered sudanophilic by heating to above their melting point during staining. Protein-bound lipid may also not be demonstrated by the simple technique as the protein restricts the entry of the hydrophobic dye. These protein-bound lipids are sometimes called masked lipids and they can still be demonstrated provided the lipid can be detached from the dye, e.g. by hydrolysis with acid.

Free fatty acids and phosphoglycerides, being more amphipathic, have a greater tendency to be extracted by the solvents used but their solubility can be reduced by bromination which also converts any cholesterol to a compound that is liquid at room temperature and so will also stain.

Sudan black

One further Sudan dye used is Sudan black. This is a mixture of two main hydrophobic dyes plus several hydrophilic components. It is a more aggressive dye mixture and will often stain lipids that are partly hydrophilic (amphipathic) and which would be left unstained by oil red O. It will unfortunately sometimes stain other tissue components as well as lipids, making interpretation more difficult. This unwanted staining increases as the dye solution ages and is less pronounced with fresh dye solutions.

A negative control for lysochrome techniques can be performed by using a section extracted with a 2:1 chloroform–methanol mixture for 1 h. The solvent will extract all the lipids and so destroy any true sudanophilia. Any coloration after the extraction will be non-specific and not lipid.

Phospholipids

These are lipids which contain a phosphate group. They are mainly phosphoglycerides and are principally associated with membranes, including the myelin sheaths of nerves. The presence of the phosphate group renders them more hydrophilic (i.e. they are amphipathic) than the neutral fats so they stain less readily with lysochrome techniques and are more rapidly and easily extracted than other lipids unless they are bound to protein.

Baker's acid haematein staining

This involves the reaction of phospholipids, especially choline-containing phospholipids, with potassium dichromate. The

The dangers of dissolving the lipid by using an organic solvent as the dye carrier led to an attempt to avoid using a solvent. The gelatine method developed by Govan used gelatine as a carrier instead. In this method the dye was originally dissolved in acetone but this was mixed with a hot solution of gelatine. The acetone evaporates, leaving the dye trapped within the colloidal suspension of the gelatine. The method does work but the slight theoretical advantage of not having any solvent present did not compensate for a complex and messy technique, and the method has not stood the test of time. A good theoretical idea does not always translate into a useful and workable method.

dichromate adds on to the lipids:

$$\underset{\overset{|}{H-C}}{\overset{\overset{|}{H-C}}{\|}} + \left[\begin{array}{c} O \diagdown \diagup O \\ Cr \\ O \diagup\diagdown O \end{array} \right]^{2-} + 2\,H \longrightarrow \underset{\overset{|}{H-C-O}}{\overset{\overset{|}{H-C-O}}{}} \diagup\diagdown Cr \underset{\diagdown OH}{\diagup OH}$$

The chromium can then act as a mordant for the haematein dye and the phospholipids stain blue. Any lipid unaffected by the dichromate will be lost during the dehydration and clearing so the reaction is reasonably selective. It is usually controlled by using a second sample which is treated with a simple solvent extraction before treatment with dichromate. The control differentiates phospholipids from tissue ions that may act as mordants. This technique, as well as being a histochemical technique, is also a good way to demonstrate mitochondria.

The original technique was a block staining method and involved prolonged exposure to all the reagents (for a total of 3–5 days) but the time involved can be reduced by using cryostat sections instead of blocks of tissue and this also makes controls more realistic since adjacent sections can be used for the test and the control.

Marchi techniques for myelin

This relies on the following properties:

- osmium tetroxide is soluble in both hydrophobic and amphipathic lipids;
- osmium tetroxide is an oxidizing agent which oxidizes and blackens lipids;
- hydrophilic oxidizing agents such as potassium dichromate or potassium chlorate are only able to penetrate amphipathic lipids;
- the oxidizing and blackening effect of osmium tetroxide is inhibited by other oxidizing agents.

So if a mixed reagent of osmium tetroxide and potassium dichromate (a hydrophilic oxidizing agent) is applied to tissues then the amphipathic lipids will absorb both the osmium tetroxide and the potassium dichromate. Since the dichromate will inhibit the blackening effect of the osmium tetroxide, the amphipathic lipids will not become blackened. The hydrophobic lipids will absorb the osmium tetroxide but not the potassium dichromate so they will become blackened. Thus the total effect is that hydrophobic lipids will be blackened but more hydrophilic or amphipathic lipids will not.

This is one way to identify degenerating myelin. Normal myelin consists of hydrophilic phospholipid while the degenerating myelin is converted to hydrophobic neutral lipid. With Marchi-type techniques normal myelin is unstained and degenerate myelin is black.

The original Marchi method used potassium dichromate but the Swank–Davenport method employing potassium chlorate is now generally preferred.

OTAN (osmium tetroxide alpha-naphthylamine)

This is similar to the Marchi-type techniques but the osmium that is bound by phospholipids but not blackened is demonstrated by using alpha-naphthylamine which gives an orange/red or orange/brown complex with the osmium. The OTAN technique has lost popularity because its specificity has been questioned (hydrophobic lipids and some proteins may also be stained) and in addition alpha-naphthylamine may be carcinogenic especially if contaminated with beta-naphthylamine.

Steroids: cholesterol

Cholesterol is the only steroid that is present in large enough amounts to be detectable in tissue sections. Large amounts of cholesterol may form crystals within the tissues and when they dissolve out in processing their presence is indicated by angular gaps in the tissues referred to as cholesterol clefts.

Cholesterol is not normally sudanophilic

Cholesterol will not be stained by the normal lysochrome technique as it has a high melting point and is crystalline at room temperature. By staining at a temperature above its melting point (150°C) it will become sudanophilic but staining at this high temperature is inconvenient. It can also be rendered sudanophilic by treatment with bromine water (2.5% aqueous bromine) when it is converted into an oily liquid that will stain with Sudan black.

The PAN method

The best specific method for cholesterol is the perchloric acid–naphthaquinone reaction (PAN). The perchloric acid converts the cholesterol to a diene that then reacts with 1,2-naphthaquinone to give a blue product. In practice the cholesterol first needs to be oxidized and this can be done using ferric chloride. The reagent also includes ethanol and formaldehyde but their exact role is not completely clear. The reaction is usually done on a hotplate at 70°C and the reagent is constantly brushed on to the section to prevent drying.

Cholesterol esters can be distinguished from free cholesterol by treating a second section with digitonin. This precipitates free cholesterol as a digitonide that is insoluble in acetone. The section is then treated with acetone. The acetone dissolves and removes the cholesterol esters but leaves the cholesterol digitonide. The PAN

Large amounts of cholesterol are found mainly in degenerating tissues such as during necrosis. The cholesterol is a normal constituent of cell membranes but is difficult for the body to remove. As tissues degenerate the cholesterol accumulates. This occurs for example when atherosclerosis occurs. The wall of an artery becomes damaged and as cells disintegrate cholesterol accumulates, partly from the degenerating cells and partly from low density lipoprotein (LDL) that carries cholesterol in the blood, and this gets trapped in the vessel wall. The lipid is ingested by macrophages which develop a foamy looking cytoplasm ('foam cells'). Repair mechanisms are activated and result in a fibrotic plaque. The lesion gets worse with time and can lead to narrowing of the arterial lumen and even complete blockage. The degeneration is slow and may even reverse if the cholesterol can be removed by **high density lipoprotein** (HDL). The full mechanism of this degeneration is still unresolved but high levels of LDL cholesterol are bad for the arteries and high levels of HDL are good for avoiding cardiovascular disease.

technique is then applied to the extracted section. Material reacting in both sections is free cholesterol whilst any material reacting in the straight PAN but absent from the digitonin-treated slide is a cholesterol ester.

Free fatty acids

Free fatty acids are unusual in normal tissues but can occur in acute pancreatitis when the release of lipases results in the fats being enzymically hydrolysed. Free fatty acids can be demonstrated by treating the section with copper salts. Any fatty acid will form insoluble copper soaps with the copper ions. The copper soaps can then be demonstrated with copper-detecting reagents such as rubeanic acid (dithio-oxamide).

In many cases the free fatty acids will have already formed calcium soaps if they have been in contact with solutions containing calcium ions. This may occur in the body or if the tissues have been fixed in formal-calcium. These calcium soaps need to be hydrolysed with hydrochloric acid before being treated with the copper ions.

Phosphatidyl ethanolamine-based lipids (plasmalogens)

Plasmalogens can be detected by the plasmal reaction (from which they get their name). This involves treatment with mercuric chloride which reacts with the vinyl ether linkage found in plasmalogens. This releases an aldehyde that can be detected using Schiff's reagent. The reaction may even occur without pretreatment of the tissues with mercuric chloride if the Schiff's reagent is highly acid and the treatment with Schiff's is prolonged since the acidity can have a similar bond-splitting effect.

Unsaturated lipids

The double bonds in lipids can be detected in a number of ways. As has already been mentioned, osmium tetroxide adds across double bonds and blackens the lipid in the process. The double bonds can also be oxidized to aldehydes and the aldehydes detected by Schiff's reagent. The oxidation can be achieved by using a powerful oxidizing agent such as performic acid (performic acid–Schiff, PFAS) but will occur slowly even with atmospheric oxygen. This slow oxidation will result in aldehydes occurring in the section without any pretreatment and is called a pseudoplasmal reaction and is a nuisance when using Schiff's reagent as it can give a non-specific background colour to the sections. The oxidation by air can be speeded up by irradiating the section with UV light and the UV Schiff technique is an alternative to using the performic acid–Schiff reaction and avoids the use of the highly corrosive performic acid.

Like cholesterol, unsaturated lipids are linked to cardiovascular disease. In this case the unsaturated lipids are protective and it is the saturated lipids that are bad. The monounsaturated olive oil is often recommended as being a good lipid and may help prevent heart disease.

Glycolipids

These will give a positive reaction with the periodic acid–Schiff technique but require controls to distinguish them from mucins and other carbohydrates. The simplest is an extraction with chloroform–methanol. There can also be confusion with plasmalogens which can give a positive reaction with Schiff's reagent and pseudoplasmal reactions.

Extraction techniques as controls and for identification

Lipids can be identified by their solubility. Extraction is a standard technique in lipid biochemistry and the difference in solubility of the different lipids forms the basis of chromatography which is the best way of identifying individual lipids. In histology the solubility of a lipid is determined by lipid staining two equivalent sections one of which has been extracted with a particular solvent. By using different solvents it is possible to selectively remove different lipids. The example given in Table 7.1 shows the method of Keilig.

The table gives a false impression of the ease and accuracy of the method, and extraction results are not easy to interpret. For example, it is usually necessary to use a Soxhlet apparatus and continuous refluxing for long periods to ensure removal of the lipid. The problems with extraction are:

- The lipid may relocalize rather than dissolve. This may be unrelated to the solvent since heating itself alters the lipid, which may move significantly during the treatment giving the impression that it has dissolved whilst it has only flowed to a different area of the tissue.

- The solubility is determined on pure lipids but in tissues the lipids are often mixtures and this can affect their solubility in solvents.

- Lipids in tissues are often intimately bound to proteins which may alter their solubility.

- Lipids in sections have often been exposed to fixatives which may affect their solubility.

In practice extraction techniques are rarely used as a major way of

As with the mucopolysaccharidoses, if there is a defect in the destruction of lipids it can lead to a disease in which lipids build up. Tay–Sach's disease (TSD) is a genetic disease in which the hexosaminidase enzyme of lysosomes is defective. This prevents the destruction of one type of glycolipid (gangliosides) which accumulate in the lysosomes. The childhood form of this disease is particularly associated with Jewish populations originating in Eastern Europe (Ashkenazi Jews). The Ashkenazi Jews have a much higher incidence of the gene in the population with perhaps as many as 1 in 25 people being a carrier of the gene compared to 1 in 500 in the general population. Affected children are therefore much commoner in these Jewish populations. The disease causes swelling of neurones which can lead to seizures, poor development and blindness. The disease begins to affect the child from about the age of 3 months and leads to death at around 4–5 years old.

Table 7.1 *Selective removal of lipids: the Keilig method*

Solvent	Lipids dissolved
Cold acetone	Glycerides, cholesterol and its esters and other steroids
Hot acetone	Cerebroside lipids
Hot ether	Lecithin and cephalins
Hot chloroform and methanol	All lipids

identifying individual lipids but they can be very useful control methods.

Suggested further reading

Bancroft, J.D. and Cook, H.C. (1994). *Manual of Histological Techniques and their Diagnostic Application.* Edinburgh: Churchill Livingstone.

BaylissHigh, O.B. and Lake, B. (1996). Lipids, in *Theory and Practice of Histological Techniques* (eds J.D. Bancroft and A. Stevens). Edinburgh: Churchill Livingstone.

Cook, H.C. (1974). *Manual of Histological Demonstration Techniques.* London: Butterworths.

Kiernan, J.A. (1990). *Histological and Histochemical Methods.* Oxford: Pergamon.

Sheehan, D.C. and Hrapchak, B. (1980). *Theory and Practice of Histotechnology.* St Louis: Mosby.

Self-assessment questions

1. What are the extra difficulties in identifying chemicals in sections compared to in solution?
2. What type of materials stain with the PAS technique?
3. Why is periodic acid preferred as the oxidizing agent compared to chromic acid or potassium permanganate?
4. List the main types of mucins.
5. Outline the principle of the critical electrolyte concentration in relation to using Alcian blue.
6. How could you distinguish between hyaluronic acid and sialic acid containing mucins, both of which stain with Alcian blue?
7. Why are lipid techniques unpopular with many histologists?
8. What is the principle of staining lipids with Sudan-type dyes?
9. Which, if any, fixatives can fix lipids?
10. Why does normal myelin react differently with lipid staining techniques compared to degenerating myelin?

Key Concepts and Facts

General Considerations

- Histochemistry is the application of chemical and biochemical techniques to tissue sections.

- Histochemistry is limited by the need to have an insoluble coloured product to localize the site of the reaction.

- Histochemistry needs careful controlling to ensure that the methods are sufficiently sensitive and sufficiently selective.

Carbohydrate Histochemistry

- The PAS reaction detects materials that contain sugars, including polysaccharides, mucins and glycoproteins.

- In the PAS reaction the periodic acid oxidizes the adjacent hydroxyl groups into aldehydes which then react with the Schiff's reagent.

- Mucins are substances that have a protein core surrounded by polysaccharide chains.

- Mucins can be acidic or neutral depending on the sugars in the chains.

- Acid mucins react with Alcian blue at an acid pH.

- Acid mucins can contain sulphate or carboxylate groups.

Lipid Histochemistry

- Lipids are difficult to retain in tissue sections as they are difficult to fix.

- Lipids are usually demonstrated in cryostat sections.

- Many lipids can be stained by using a hydrophobic dye in aqueous solution (lysochromic staining).

- Specific tests are available to distinguish the main types of lipid.

Chapter 8
Histochemistry of nucleic acids, proteins and enzymes

Learning objectives

After studying this chapter you should confidently be able to:

Describe the methods of staining nucleic acids in sections.

Discuss the problems associated with identifying the type of nucleic acid.

Outline the problems associated with identifying and localizing proteins in tissue sections.

Describe the main methods for identifying proteins in sections.

Discuss the difficulties of retaining enzyme activity in sections.

Describe examples of methods for demonstrating hydrolase, dehydrogenase and oxidase enzymes.

Outline the problems involved in quantifying enzyme activity in sections.

Nucleic acids

The general structure of the nucleic acids is a backbone of alternating pentose sugar and phosphate groups. Each sugar has a nitrogenous base attached to it. The base can be either a purine or a pyrimidine. The backbone can interact with similar nucleic acid strands to form double strands by hydrogen bonding between the purine and pyrimidine bases. There are four different bases that can occur in any nucleic acid and the sequence of these bases is the basis of the genetic code. Nucleic acids include several quite different forms of material that differ in their chemical composition and structural forms.

DNA and RNA

DNA and RNA are chemically and structurally different

Ribonucleic acid (RNA) has a simple ribose sugar in the main backbone of the molecule while deoxyribonucleic acid (DNA) has the deoxyribose form of the sugar in its backbone. They differ slightly in their bases such that DNA includes the base thymine whilst RNA uses uracil in the same position. In both forms the other three bases are the same (adenine, guanine and cytosine).

DNA is found almost exclusively in the nucleus (very small amounts are found in the mitochondria) and whilst all the RNA is actually produced inside the nucleus it is usually quickly transported into the cytoplasm so that most of the RNA is found in the cytoplasm or in the nucleolus which produces the ribosomal RNA.

Probably the most important differences in the properties of the nucleic acids from a histochemical point of view are the size of the molecule, the shape of the molecule and whether there is any attached protein.

DNA double helix

DNA forms a rigid double helix and is strongly associated with histone proteins. This combination forms nucleoprotein and is the material usually referred to by histologists as chromatin. The DNA is wrapped around the histones and each structure forms a characteristic unit called a nucleosome. The DNA in a cell usually forms very large molecules with each chromosome being a single DNA molecule. So an average human chromosome consists of around 1×10^8 nucleotides and the DNA helix would measure about 5 cm if straightened out completely. The wrapping around the histones reduces this to around 1 mm in total length and more coiling and folding reduce it even further. So the DNA within the cell is always highly coiled.

Active and inert DNA

Depending on how compactly it is packed the DNA is described as being heterochromatic (darkly staining and very tightly packed) or euchromatic (lighter staining and less densely packed). Hetero-chromatin is inactive and not transcribed whilst euchromatin is being actively used by the cell. The DNA may also be modified by being methylated. In methylation some of the cytosine bases are changed to 5-methyl cytosine. This conversion is catalysed by enzymes. Methylation is believed to be a method of controlling gene activity since inactive genes tend to be more heavily methylated.

The DNA in the cell is not all used and some DNA does not seem to be used by any cell at any time. This unused DNA is referred to as non-coding DNA or is sometimes called 'junk DNA' as it serves no useful purpose and apparently clutters up the cell. It is estimated that only about 1% of the genome is actually directly used. The remainder may play a structural role in the cell or have some function we have not yet found.

About 30% of the DNA is in the form of highly repetitive sequences of DNA which may be repeated hundreds of times in the cell. At the end of each chromosome is a telomere that consists of repeats of the same sequence of bases. At cell division there is usually a loss of one telomere repeat because the copying mechanism does not fully copy the ends of the DNA. So at each cell division the telomere shortens by one repeat. Eventually it becomes so short that DNA polymerase is unable to bind to the DNA and the cell can no longer divide. This may be the cause of the so-called **Hayflick limit** where cells have a limited number of divisions before becoming senescent and dying.

Different forms of RNA

RNA comes in several different forms within the cell:

- Ribosomal RNA (rRNA). The rRNA does not form a double helix and is always associated with protein. These units form the small structures called ribosomes. Although too small to be adequately resolved as individual structures by the light microscope the ribosomes can form larger aggregates (polyribosomes) which can be visible in the cytoplasm.
- Transfer RNA (tRNA). tRNA does not form a double helix but forms a series of hairpin loops of RNA. Transfer RNA is not bound to protein.
- Messenger RNA (mRNA). mRNA does not form a double helix but occurs as a single-stranded RNA and is not firmly bound to protein.

The differences in function of the three forms of RNA are of only minor importance in most histological investigations since all three forms of RNA are associated in different ways with the production of protein. So for most histological purposes they are all indicators of active protein synthesis and, provided any one of them is retained, the loss of the other forms is less critical. It is only when mRNA is needed in hybridization studies (Chapter 13) that it is essential to retain a particular kind of RNA.

Fixation affects either the physical or chemical structure of nucleic acids

In paraffin sections only nucleic acid that is firmly attached to protein will be consistently retained since most fixatives act on proteins and not nucleic acid. This means that only DNA and rRNA are retained by all fixatives and can always be demonstrated in tissues. Some fixatives, whilst not truly fixing the nucleic acid, may still alter it either chemically or physically.

Additive fixatives usually combine with and alter the reactive groups of nucleic acids whilst non-additive fixatives alter the double helix regions of DNA and so disturb its physical form. There is no fixative that retains both the chemical and physical form of nucleic acids. Some staining methods rely on chemical reactivity whilst others use physical form to trap the dyes. Whenever nucleic acids are to be investigated it is essential to employ a fixative that retains the particular characteristic of the nucleic acid used in the demonstration method.

Generally acetic acid-containing fixatives give better preservation and are preferred for DNA studies but formaldehyde is satisfactory for DNA and rRNA.

Staining techniques

The commonest staining methods for nucleic acid involve the basic dyes. Nucleic acids are strongly basophilic and will stain with almost any basic dye. This is fine for morphological purposes but basophilia is not limited to nucleic acids and needs controlling with enzymes in order to get specific identification.

Feulgen technique

The Feulgen technique is specific for DNA and will not stain RNA. The technique uses Schiff's reagent which, as pointed out above, reacts with aldehydes. The DNA in tissues does not contain any free aldehydes but aldehydes can be produced by acid hydrolysis. The hydrolysis removes the bases from the DNA leaving sugars that contain aldehyde groups and therefore stain pink with the Schiff's reagent.

The hydrolysis of DNA is usually done with 1 M HCl at 60°C. Care must be taken to get the timing of the hydrolysis correct or the DNA will be completely hydrolysed to soluble fragments of nucleic acid and these will wash out of the section and staining will be reduced. RNA is completely hydrolysed by the usual hydrolysis and does not stain.

When the Feulgen technique is correctly performed it is quantitative and the amount of DNA in each cell can be measured by microdensitometry. The amount of DNA in an individual cell is usually constant in most human cells except when:

- The cell is actively dividing. Before division can occur the cell must duplicate the DNA so that when the cell splits into two both daughter cells will get a complete set of chromosomes.
- The cell has an unusual chromosome number.

Both of these situations are associated with malignant cells so investigations are currently underway to determine if an automatic technique can be developed which will reliably identify malignant cells by measuring their DNA content.

The Feulgen hydrolysis step is dependent on the fixative used. Picric acid performs the same hydrolysis as HCl and so picric acid fixed material is not suitable for the Feulgen technique nor is tissue decalcified in acid solutions.

The following are the optimum times for some fixatives: formaldehyde 8 min; Carnoy 8 min; Helly 5 min; SUSA 18 min. If there is as little as 30 s error in the timing then the results will be less than optimal and will be non-quantitative.

Fluorescent stains

There are a number of very valuable fluorescent dyes that can be

Although the amount of DNA within any species is constant there does not appear to be any relationship between the number of chromosomes or the amount of DNA in a species and its complexity or its need for enzymes. Humans with 3×10^9 nucleotides and 23 chromosome pairs are far from having the most DNA. Some newts have over 10 times more DNA per cell than humans and some plants have hundreds of chromosome pairs.

used to demonstrate nucleic acids. These dyes include quinacrine, Hoechst 33258, ethidium bromide and acridine orange.

Fluorescence with certain dyes is due to intercalation in the double helix

These dyes act by intercalating into nucleic acids. Intercalation is where the dye slides between the stacks of bases and is dependent on the double helix structure. Quinacrine, Hoechst 33258 and ethidium bromide are only used to stain DNA and can be used as vital stains to show DNA in living cells. Quinacrine has been used to demonstrate chromosome bands (so-called q-banding) in the identification of chromosomal structure and the diagnosis of chromosome disorders. This is because it produces bright fluorescence in adenine/thymine-rich regions and less fluorescence in guanine/cytosine-rich regions. When quin-acrine is used on the compacted chromosomes found in mitosis it gives a banding pattern of bright and dim transverse bands. The non-fluorescent dark bands represent regions rich in guanine and cytosine whilst the brighter fluorescent bands represent regions rich in adenine and thymine.

Acridine orange stains DNA and RNA

Acridine orange is different to the previous dyes in that it can be used for both DNA and RNA. With acridine orange double-stranded DNA fluoresces green whilst single-stranded RNA fluoresces red. Since it depends on the conformation of the DNA strands to distinguish the two types of nucleic acid it follows that any treatment that alters the structure will destroy this differentiation. Formaldehyde fixed and paraffin processed materials do not work reliably with this technique but it has been used on alcohol fixed smears.

Methyl green–pyronin technique

The methyl green–pyronin technique uses two different basic dyes to stain the different nucleic acids and distinguish DNA and RNA. In some ways it is the equivalent of the van Gieson or trichrome methods of using acid dyes. The dyes used are methyl green, a triaryl methane dye, and pyronin Y, a xanthene dye. The dyes differ in molecular weight, molecular size and molecular shape. When used at pH 4.6 they compete for binding to the nucleic acids and differentially stain the DNA a green colour whilst the RNA stains red.

The mechanism of this differential staining is disputed. It seems likely that the methyl green stains by binding to the outside of the DNA helix and is bound by the phosphate groups and possibly by linking non-ionically to the protein and sugars. The pyronin, being a smaller more planar molecule, can probably intercalate between the bases and stain nucleic acids in this way. The differences in

The identification of RNA by pyronin is referred to as pyroninophilia. The term is applied to cells such as the lymphoblasts and plasma cells that are active in the production of antibodies. The presence of nucleic acids in the cytoplasm can be indicated by cytoplasmic basophilia. The term pyroninophilia is more limited and refers only to nucleic acids whereas basophilia refers to any acidic material in the cytoplasm.

enzyme. This is due to the fact that the usual Beer–Lambert relationship is not necessarily applicable. In the absence of the Beer–Lambert relationship it is difficult or impossible to relate the density of colour to the activity of the enzyme.

The problems associated with quantifying enzymes in tissue sections include:

- Loss of enzyme activity in fixation, cutting etc. All processing of tissues, even just preparing frozen sections, can involve significant losses of activity. The actual amount of enzyme activity in a section is always less than was present in the original tissue.

- The rate of an enzyme's activity in a section may be controlled by how rapidly the substrate diffuses into the tissue not the amount of enzyme present. The diffusion of substrate can be effectively one-dimensional, with all the substrate coming directly down on to the site of the enzyme. Diffusion from the side will always be slower but may be non-existent if there are adjacent enzyme sites and, of course, diffusion from below is not possible since sections are normally attached to an impermeable glass slide or coverslip. If the rate of diffusion is slower than the maximal activity of the enzyme then the amount of colour produced will not follow the usual Beer–Lambert law and enzyme activity will be under-estimated.

- Diffusion rate may be altered by the precipitation of insoluble product. The nature of histochemical demonstration requires the production of an insoluble product at the site of activity. This makes the diffusion process even worse. There may be a maximum colour that can ever develop where diffusion is completely blocked, so again Beer–Lambert relationships are not valid.

- Section thickness may not be constant. This is a major problem since section thickness determines how much enzyme is present. If the thickness of sections from a microtome fluctuates by only 1 μm (1/1000 of a mm) then it may alter the thickness by as much as 20 or 25% (a nominal 5 μm section could in reality be anywhere between 4 and 6 μm). Section thickness is very difficult to measure and fluctuation in section thickness is a common finding. Sections can be alternately thicker and thinner than the set thickness. This may be due to a slightly loose knife or block or due to wear in the microtome producing looseness.

- Diffusional losses of reaction product. If the final product is even slightly soluble in any of the reagents used in processing the section then some of the colour will be lost.

Suggested further reading

Bancroft, J.D. and Cook, H.C. (1994). *Manual of Histological*

Techniques and their Diagnostic Application. Edinburgh: Churchill Livingstone.

BaylissHigh, O.B. and Lake, B. (1996). Carbohydrates, in *Theory and Practice of Histological Techniques* (eds J.D. Bancroft and A. Stevens). Edinburgh: Churchill Livingstone.

Kiernan, J.A. (1990). *Histological and Histochemical Methods.* Oxford: Pergamon.

Sheehan, D.C. and Hrapchak, B. (1980). *Theory and Practice of Histotechnology.* St Louis: Mosby.

Self-assessment questions

1. How can the basophilic staining of nuclei be controlled to ensure that it is due to DNA and not to other basophilic materials?
2. What is meant by 'intercalation'?
   Name one dye which stains by intercalation.
3. Outline the principle of the Feulgen technique.
4. Give two different ways that proteins can be stained in tissue sections and indicate how specific they are.
5. Name two ways in which enzyme activity may be lost in tissue sections.
6. What is the reason for adding potassium cyanide to substrate solutions being used to demonstrate dehydrogenase enzymes?
7. How is the naphthol azo-coupling method modified to demonstrate hydrolases other than phosphatases?
8. Why is it better to measure enzyme activity biochemically than histochemically?

Key Concepts and Facts

Nucleic Acids

- DNA and RNA are basophilic and can both be demonstrated by basic dyes. DNA can be specifically stained using the Feulgen technique.

- RNA and DNA can be distinguished using selective dyeing methods such as methyl green–pyronin or by using enzyme digestion.

Proteins

- Most proteins are acidophilic and will stain with acid dyes.

- Only a few proteins can be identified by simple staining methods.

- The amino acids in proteins can be demonstrated but this is not commonly done.

- Individual proteins are best demonstrated by immunological methods.

Enzymes

- Enzymes are a special group of proteins that can be demonstrated by their catalytic activity.

- Only hydrolytic and oxidative enzymes are commonly demonstrated in tissues.

- Tissues must be cut fresh since fixation will destroy enzyme activity.

Chapter 9

Histochemistry of pigments, neuroendocrine amines and minerals

Learning objectives

After studying this chapter you should confidently be able to:

Describe the main types of pigment found in sections.

Outline the tests used in identifying pigments.

Describe the formalin-induced fluorescence reaction of neuro-endocrine amines.

List the main minerals found in tissue sections and describe how they can be identified.

Outline the use of ion selective dyes.

The pigments discussed in the main text are the common ones encountered in tissue sections but other pigments do occasionally occur but are rarely demonstrated.

The slight yellow colour of fat is due to fat soluble plant pigments such as carotenoids. These pigments are of no significance in the usual amounts and I have only heard of one person who was adversely affected. He was highly exceptional and died of vitamin A overdose. He was taking vitamin A tablets and drinking lots of carrot juice and he went quite a bright orange colour. Most people don't suffer from the small amounts present in their bodies.

Pigments

Most materials in tissue sections are uncoloured until a stain is applied but a few materials are coloured and can be seen in unstained sections. These self-coloured materials are referred to as pigments. They include a wide variety of materials from different sources and have differing significance. The presence of some pigments is normal but others can be related to disease and so it is often important to be able to recognize and identify them.

When identifying pigments two features need to be borne in mind about the appearance and reactions of the materials.

- Firstly, the materials generally have a limited range of colour with most being yellow to brown or brown to black. The colour varies depending on how much is present. A brown pigment present as a very heavy deposit may appear almost black whilst the same pigment present in only small amounts may appear yellowish. Thus descriptions of the colour are only a **guide** and **not a precise description**.

- Secondly, the results of a test are affected by the colour of the pigment. Schmorl's test for example gives a blue colour as a positive reaction but if it is applied to a yellow pigment then a positive result will be greenish (blue + yellow) rather than pure blue. This also means that it may be difficult to see if a reaction has occurred. How can you tell what has happened if a positive reaction gives a black colour but the pigment is already black?

Pigments can be conveniently grouped into three major types with one type being further subdivided. These groups are merely convenient labels and some pigments can be put into more than one category:

- artefact pigments;
- exogenous pigments;
- endogenous pigments – haematogenous and autogenous.

Artefact pigments

These are not originally part of the tissue but have been added by the processes used to prepare the tissue. The commonest are associated with fixatives as follows.

Formalin (formaldehyde) pigment

Formaldehyde pigment is most easily seen around old or degenerating blood in tissues fixed in acid solutions of formaldehyde. Most of the pigment is easily prevented by using buffered formaldehyde for fixation. The pigment appears as a fine brownish deposit around the old blood. Formaldehyde pigment can be identified and removed by treatment with picric acid solutions.

Mercury pigment

This is a dense black, granular (or occasionally globular) pigment, occurring irregularly throughout the tissue. It cannot be prevented if the fixative contains mercuric chloride but it is easily removed by treating the section with iodine solutions (this also acts as a test to recognize mercury though all heavy metal derived pigments will also be dissolved). Mercury pigment is less common in modern histological practice where mercury-containing fixatives are less used, but is found in tissues stored in archives as mercuric chloride was once a very common fixative.

Chrome pigment

This pigment may be found as a brownish pigment in tissues fixed in chrome fixatives and not washed out in water before processing. It occurs when the chrome salt reacts with the alcohols used in tissue processing and produces a brown oxide, though the reaction is not easily produced even when it is done deliberately as a demonstration. Chrome pigment is not easily removed once formed so it is better to avoid it by always washing out chromium-fixed tissues in water.

Osmium pigment

This occurs as a very dense black pigment spread throughout the tissue following fixation in osmium tetroxide (commonly used for EM specimens). It is not usually a problem since in EM it acts as a stain and when it is used in light microscopy the blackening is often used to identify double bonds. However, it can be removed from sections by oxidation with hydrogen peroxide if this is needed for some stains.

Exogenous pigments

Exogenous pigments were present in the original tissue but are not a normal part of the body and are contaminants that entered the body during life. The pigments are either ingested, inhaled or otherwise introduced in life. The significance varies, with some being pathological and some indicators of the person's employment (e.g. silica) or their lifestyle (e.g. tattoos).

Carbon

Carbon usually occurs as a dense black pigment. Carbon may be intracellular in macrophages when it is often seen as a fine powder or can occur in angular clumps in the extracellular connective tissue. Carbon is very common in the lungs of city dwellers and more especially smokers. It also occurs in regional lymph nodes around the lungs where it has been carried by macrophages. Less commonly it can sometimes be seen in skin from tattoos and needle tracks. The carbon itself is not pathological though the association with tobacco smoke does have links with smoking-related disease.

Carbon is difficult to identify accurately as it is very inert. Usually it can be reliably identified by its location (lungs) and shape. It can be destroyed by microincineration but this is not commonly done. It has no pathological significance in itself but it sometimes needs to be distinguished from other black pigments that may be important. This can be done by eliminating the other pigments by testing for each one in turn.

Silica

This may be brown to black in colour depending on the source of the silica and is found as angular masses in the lungs and lymph

A variety of pigments are sometimes used in tattoos. Carbon is one that sometimes occurs especially in 'amateur tattoos'. In professional tattoos the pigments used can be much more elaborate and of many different colours. The pigments don't usually need to be identified but if you wish to see the colours then use an incident-light microscope rather than the usual transmitted-light microscope.

Protein coating   Asbestos fibre   **Figure 9.1** *Asbestos body*

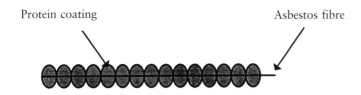

nodes of miners, quarry workers, stonemasons and other people exposed to stone dust especially from power grinding equipment.

Silica is very inert as it is the same material as glass, and it is difficult to identify with specific tests. There are no positive tests and it is unaffected by all histochemical reagents and microincineration. Silica may be birefringent (rotates the plane of polarized light) and may show brightly using a polarizing microscope, and this is often a useful indicator.

Silica causes the disease silicosis which is a serious and often fatal fibrosis of the lungs. Silicosis is a recognized industrial disease so that assessment of the amount of damage caused by silica may be important in cases of industrial compensation.

Asbestos

This occurs as a brown pigment found in the lungs but usually appearing as fibres rather than the angular masses associated with silica. Inside the body it becomes coated in an iron-containing protein that forms distinctive beaded asbestos bodies (Figure 9.1). The asbestos bodies are easily recognized and give a positive Perls reaction for iron.

The fibres are inert and birefringent (the different types of asbestos can be identified by their birefringence). As with silica, asbestos is not destroyed by microincineration. Asbestos is often associated with disease and it causes asbestosis which can be very debilitating and is a recognized industrial disease. Asbestos increases the risk of developing lung cancer and is the only known cause of the malignant mesothelioma tumour.

Silica causes the damage to cells by its ability to form hydrogen bonds with membranes. If very fine particles get into the lungs they will be ingested by macrophages and end up in the lysosomes. Here the silica particles can hydrogen bond to the lysosomal membrane and cause it to rupture. The lysosomal enzymes are released into the cytoplasm and kill the cell. The enzymes break down both the cell and surrounding tissue. The silica is inert and it remains unaffected. The silica will be ingested by another macrophage and the cycle will be repeated. This results in a chronic inflammation and scar tissue forms where there tissue is damaged. The cycle will continue to repeat until the silica becomes coated with enough protein or fibrous tissue for it to be ignored by macrophages. If the silica load in the lungs is big then large areas of the lungs will become replaced by fibrous scar tissue and this is the cause of silicosis.

Endogenous pigments

Endogenous pigments are the products of metabolism in the body. They occur naturally within the tissues and so occur in normal tissues. They are, however, also associated with disease states when they occur in excessive amounts or in unusual situations. The pigments can come from blood or one of its breakdown products (haematogenous pigments) or be derived from other metabolic processes (autogenous pigments).

Haematogenous pigments

These are all derived from the blood in one way or another.

Haemoglobin

This is always present in the tissues inside the red blood cells (RBCs) and in this form it is usually ignored as a pigment. It does, however, sometimes occur outside the RBCs, for example in haemolytic diseases, and then it becomes significant. Haemoglobin has a molecular size that is close to the limit of the glomerular filtration system. Once haemoglobin is released into the plasma it can pass through the glomerular filter into the renal tubules and this can lead to renal problems.

Haemoglobin in formalin fixed sections is not the bright red colour usually associated with blood but is a brownish colour. Free haemoglobin is an amorphous or globular material that is strongly acidophilic. Haemoglobin can be identified by this strong acidophilia. The eosin in a haematoxylin and eosin stain gives a more orange-pink colour to haemoglobin than to other materials in the section and this is often sufficiently distinctive to allow haemoglobin to be identified, but more specialized techniques have been developed, e.g. the almond green/kiton red stain, which give an even better distinction.

Histochemically haemoglobin can be identified by the peroxidase activity of the haemoglobin molecule (see Chapter 8 for the peroxidase reaction). This peroxidase activity is unusual in that it resists normal processing and can often be demonstrated in paraffin wax sections.

Haemosiderin and ferritin

A whole range of iron-binding proteins occurs in cells and tissues to scavenge and recycle the iron released by the degradation of haemoglobin. Many are present in such small quantities that they cannot be easily visualized by light microscopy. Larger deposits occur as brown granular or powdery deposits, particularly in macrophages of the spleen and liver (where destruction of old RBCs occurs) and around sites of haemorrhage. These larger accumulations are called haemosiderin by histologists. Haemosiderin is easily identified by the Perls reaction which detects the iron in the haemosiderin. The iron is detected by potassium ferrocyanide [potassium hexacyanoferrate(III)]. This produces a dense blue precipitate (the pigment Prussian blue; hence the other names for the test, Prussian blue reaction, PBR, or Perls Prussian blue reaction, PPBR).

The iron in haemosiderin will not react directly with the ferrocyanide but must be released from the protein by acid hydrolysis. So the Perls reagent is a mixture of 2% potassium ferrocyanide and 2% hydrochloric acid. The iron in haemoglobin is too strongly held within the porphyrin ring to be released in this way and so haemoglobin and RBCs are Perls-negative.

Other tests are available for haemosiderin (Turnbull's blue and blackening of the free iron with hydrogen sulphide) but are rarely used.

Diseases associated with excess haemosiderin include haemochromatosis and haemosiderosis. It is also an important way of identifying sites of tissue damage (remnants of bleeding) and identification of haemosiderin is useful in identifying some types of cells.

Bile pigments

These are derived from the porphyrin ring of haemoglobin. They vary in colour from red-brown (bilirubin, the commonest form) to greens (biliverdin). The range of colours seen in a bruise as it heals is mainly due to the breakdown of these pigments. Bile pigments are slightly soluble in organic solvents so small amounts are usually lost and paraffin sections of normal liver cells (the main site of pigment production) are usually free from pigment. Only large deposits can resist processing and appear in wax sections.

Bile pigments are difficult to identify. They can be identified by oxidation which alters the colour. The Fouchet technique uses ferric chloride as an oxidant in the presence of trichloracetic acid. This gives a bright green colour which is fairly stable but not all forms of bile pigment will react.

Gmelin's test uses concentrated nitric acid as the oxidizing agent and reacts with more types of bile pigment but the colour change is fleeting. Sections are examined whilst the test is being applied but even so the colour changes can easily be missed and the slides cannot be kept or viewed later. A positive result is usually reliable but a negative result with the normal tests should not be considered conclusive. The test involves oxidation of the pigments by irrigation. This means running the reagent under the coverslip whilst viewing the section. The reagents are quite corrosive and the difficulties of looking down the microscope and focusing on the section at the same time as squeezing nitric acid out of a Pasteur pipette mean that it is a cumbersome technique and is best carried out using three arms and two heads. For most people this means getting someone else to help while you do the test.

Excessive amounts of bile pigment are found in some liver diseases or in haemolytic disease.

Autogenous pigments

This group of pigments is in many ways quite diverse and contains pigments derived from metabolism but not associated directly with blood. Despite their diverse origin they do have one common

In melanosis coli the gut becomes almost black due to the accumulation of a pigment in the macrophages similar to lipofuscin. This condition is caused by excessive use of purgative laxatives. Despite the name the pigment is not related to melanin and it is just the sheer amount of pigment that causes the dark colour. The pigment is sometimes called pseudomelanin.

characteristic. They are all reducing pigments. This makes them a neat group in practice since a single reducing test allows them to be identified as belonging to this group.

Two reducing tests are in use:

- Masson–Fontana silver reduction (black result);
- Schmorl's ferricyanide reduction (blue result).

The first is more sensitive but is slow (24 h or more) and the black result may be difficult to interpret if the pigment itself is dark brown or black. The Schmorl's test is quicker (5–15 min) but is often difficult to interpret because the background tissue takes on a greenish tinge.

Melanin

This is a black or brown pigment that is found in the eye (especially the retina), skin (especially negroid skin, tanned skin and around the nipples) and in parts of the brain (substantia nigra). Melanin can be identified by its reducing ability with Schmorl's, appearance and the fact that it is bleached by oxidizing agents (hydrogen peroxide, potassium permanganate or potassium chlorate/HCl).

The main pathological significance of melanin is its association with malignant melanoma.

Lipofuscin

This is a pigment derived from oxidized lipid. It appears as droplets in the lysosomes of cells. It accumulates with age and is sometimes called 'wear and tear' pigment. It is increased after some poisons (e.g. carbon tetrachloride) and in some chronic diseases. It can be found in any tissue but is often prominent in heart muscle, liver and brain.

Lipofuscin is the most easily identified of the autogenous pigments as there are several good tests which, whilst individually not conclusive, become highly selective when two or three are used in combination:

- It is basophilic; methylene blue and aldehyde fuchsin both give good strong staining.
- It is PAS-positive but this is less useful as there are many other materials in the tissues that are also PAS-positive. However, it is useful to remember that this may be the cause of an unidentified PAS-positive reaction.
- It stains as a lipid with some fat soluble dyes especially Sudan black.
- It is PAAS- and PFAS-positive (typical of unsaturated lipid) though since these are dangerous methods I would always use a simpler and safer technique.

- It stains positive by the ZN technique. This is usually used for the acid-fast mycobacteria associated with TB and leprosy but is a useful method for lipofuscin.

Chromaffin pigment

This is a brownish intracellular pigment that is found in adrenaline producing cells (adrenal medulla and sympathetic ganglia). The pigment is not entirely natural as it only occurs after an oxidizing fixative such as chrome fixatives (hence the name, from 'chrome affinity') and is not seen in formaldehyde fixed tissues. Chromaffin pigment represents the oxidized precursor of adrenaline.

It is often considered not to be a pigment since it is a part of the normal metabolism and it can be considered along with the other neurotransmitter amines and demonstrated by the formalin-induced fluorescent (FIF) technique on freeze-dried tissue. It can also be considered as an artefact pigment since it only occurs after fixation in chrome fixatives and is not a natural pigment. However, it has traditionally been included as a pigment and has been retained in this section as it is often easier to demonstrate it by fixing a piece of tissue in a chrome fixative than to do a full FIF on freeze-dried tissue. It is a basophilic pigment and gives green colour when stained with Giemsa.

Excessive chromaffin is found in phaeochromocytomas which are tumours of the chromaffin or adrenaline secreting tissues.

Argentaffin

This pigment is the strongest reducing pigment and will react strongly with silver reagents (hence its name). It is found in the endocrine secreting cells of the gut (argentaffin cells). It again only occurs after certain fixatives particularly formaldehyde and is strongly fluorescent (formalin-induced fluorescence or FIF; see below). It also reacts with diazo salts such as fast red B giving a flame-red deposit. Argentaffin pigment also gives a chromaffin reaction if fixed in chrome fixatives and can be called enterochromaffin pigment (hence the alternative name for argentaffin cells is enterochromaffin or EC cells).

Other pigments also occur but are less commonly encountered (e.g. ochronosis pigment) and will not be considered here.

Neuroendocrine granules

The neuroendocrine cells are a scattered group of cells which secrete biologically active amines as hormones. These amines are more commonly thought of as neurotransmitters but in these cells they are secreted into the bloodstream rather than into the synapses between nerve cells. They also secrete characteristic neuropeptides

The neuroendocrine cells form a useful system but their embryonic origin and relationship to each other is disputed. They may not even all come from the same original embryonic layer but the difficulty of tracing cells as they migrate in embryonic development means that no one is certain of their origin.

They form a coherent set of cells in functional terms and also have a characteristic set of tumours, APUDomas, which continue to secrete their peptides and can result in clinical syndromes due to this secretion. Carcinoid tumours are tumours arising from the gut or respiratory tract APUD cells but do not secrete any identifiable peptide hormone.

Although the biogenic amines are difficult to demonstrate in tissues they are very important in disease. They play a crucial role in the inflammatory response. Mast cells are the main cells producing these amines but the amines that are present vary with species. Human mast cells, like all mammalian mast cells, contain histamine, but rat mast cells also contain serotonin and ruminant mast cells contain dopamine.

that act as hormones. The set of cells is also known as the 'diffuse endocrine system' and the APUD system (Amine Precursor Uptake and Decarboxylation) from their metabolic activity. The amines are formed by the decarboxylation of precursor materials such as tryptophan to form serotonin (5-hydroxytryptamine or 5-HT).

Staining techniques for neuropeptides

The neuropeptide secretions are reasonably well preserved in fixed sections and can usually be stained using dyeing techniques. There are many quite selective methods that will stain different cells within the same neuroendocrine organ in different colours. Methods for the pituitary and pancreas are available to distinguish the main cell types on the basis of their acidophilic and basophilic character. These stains are usually quite attractive with clear, bright colours, but require a fair degree of skill to get good results. These methods are largely empirical and so do not have any particular theoretical interest. The peptides can also be specifically demonstrated by using immunotechniques. The main interest in neuropeptide identification involves their role in the diagnosis of tumours of the diffuse endocrine system.

Demonstrating neuroendocrine amines

The other secretory components of the neuroendocrine cells are much more difficult to demonstrate because of their low molecular weight and solubility. Materials such as adrenaline and histamine are usually lost during processing as they readily diffuse and are quickly destroyed by enzymes. The only efficient way to preserve the amines is to freeze-dry the tissues. The snap-freezing prevents diffusion and subliming away the water prevents their loss. Some amines can be detected in routine paraffin sections if they are bound to a larger tissue component. This seems to occur with serotonin (5-HT) in argentaffin cells (and rat mast cells) and with histamine in mast cell granules.

Individual methods for some materials

One or two demonstration methods have developed to show individual amines. The specificity of some of these methods is not very high but they can be useful for tumours to demonstrate that a material is present. An example of this is the silver reduction by argentaffin cells. The method is not specific for the serotonin in these cells but is a useful histological method and can be helpful in the recognition of carcinoid tumours. Similarly you can use the chromaffin method for catecholamines in the adrenal medulla using an oxidizing fixative to preserve the adrenaline and noradrenaline. Serotonin can also be demonstrated using an azo-coupling method which reacts with the phenolic group of the serotonin.

Fluorescent product with formaldehyde

The amines will react with formaldehyde to give a fluorescent product. This is the formalin-induced fluorescent technique (FIF). The reaction does not occur readily in solution (the amines will rapidly diffuse away) and instead it must be done on freeze-dried sections using formaldehyde vapour. The tissues are freeze-dried and then transferred to a closed container along with some paraformaldehyde and heated to generate formaldehyde vapour. The temperature and humidity are critical factors for maximum fluorescence and may need to be slightly altered to adjust for differences in tissues and preparation. Generally a temperature of between 60 and 80°C for 1 h is used at a relative humidity of 50–75%.

The tissue can then be embedded in paraffin wax. This does not need any processing since the tissue is freeze-dried; simply put the tissue in molten wax and gently reduce the pressure to remove air bubbles. The tissue can be blocked-out and sectioned, but water must be avoided so they are not floated on a water bath to flatten them. The tissue is dewaxed, but not rehydrated, and mounted under a coverslip. The fluorescence can be seen if the specimens are irradiated with blue-violet light of 410 nm wavelength. Dopamine and noradrenaline fluoresce green whilst serotonin gives a yellower colour.

Glyoxylic acid can replace formaldehyde

Instead of using formaldehyde a similar reaction can be produced using glyoxylic acid. The glyoxylic acid can be used to perfuse the animal, thus generating a weakly fluorescent compound before removing the tissue from the animal. Glyoxylic acid will react with cryostat sections and this is more convenient than the block method used for FIF and can give a brighter result. The fluorescence is intensified by heating or treating with formaldehyde vapour. The sensitivity of this method is very great and it has been estimated that 10^{-7} picomoles of adrenaline can be detected in cells.

Other fluorescent methods

Although formaldehyde and glyoxylic acid are the most used forms of induced fluorescence it is possible to get condensation reactions with other materials such as o-phthalaldehyde (histamine), hydrochloric acid (dopamine), acetaldehyde, glutaraldehyde and acetic acid (similar to FIF).

FIF and related methods have been mainly used in research to identify and locate the nerves using the amine neurotransmitters. FIF has been replaced to some extent by antibody techniques using antibodies against the enzymes producing the amines. This is more convenient as routine paraffin sections can be used, but these

Metals are extremely important in metabolism and there are a huge number of 'trace elements' which are needed by the body, but these are often in such minute quantities that there is no method sensitive enough to detect them in single sections. These include elements such as cobalt (found in vitamin B_{12}) and zinc (found in zinc finger structures of proteins).

Many metals are also poisonous, but even in toxic amounts they may still be difficult to demonstrate histochemically. Some metals only ever seem to be toxic, e.g. cadmium, mercury and lead. The role of other materials is less certain, for example arsenic which is certainly highly toxic, yet some evidence exists that it may be used by the metabolism but only in minute amounts.

methods only show which cells are producing amines and not how much is present. In some cases it is useful to detect which nerves are depleted of their transmitters as well as which ones are capable of producing the transmitters. The depletion can only be seen using FIF or a related method.

Metals and their compounds

The histochemistry of metals and their salts is partly dependent on their solubility. In most cases of sectioned material the only metallic materials that are likely to be present are those that are insoluble. The metal-containing compounds can be roughly divided into four different types:

- elemental metals;
- soluble metal salts;
- insoluble metal salts;
- organically bound metals.

Elemental metals

Elemental metals are found as the solid element and not combined with any other material. Such metals are uncommon in sections except as contaminants or exogenous implants. Metals are used in medicine in the form of dental fillings, radiotherapy implants and metal prostheses such as replacement joints, pins and plates in bones, and metal implants in arteries used to open out the narrowing lumens ('stents'). Identification of the materials is rarely a problem in these cases. Preparing sections of these materials, however, can be extremely difficult. Radiotherapy implants may be left in place permanently and the tissues may not be removed until much later. They can ruin a knife edge if they are unwittingly left in the paraffin wax block and may rip through the tissues, at the same time damaging the tissue itself. Occasionally sections are required, usually for research, with the implant in place and the tissue still adhering to it. Depending on the metals used, sectioning can be near to impossible but histochemical identification is not a problem.

Soluble metal salts

The soluble metal salts will be ionic and are not able to be demonstrated or localized in sections produced by any method since they will be rapidly either lost or relocated by any technique. Metal salts are ionic and very mobile. Simply cutting the tissues will allow them to diffuse. Frozen sections are not necessarily any better since the section often thaws briefly during cutting and then refreezes, and relocation could occur in that brief instant. Even freeze-drying may not prevent movement since the salts may be soluble in wax or plastic monomers. It may sometimes be possible to precipitate the metal by some means but even then relocation is more likely than accurate localization. The only method of localizing these materials is to examine intact living cells without sectioning using ion-sensitive dyes (see below) but this is not always a reasonable method to apply.

Insoluble metal salts

The insoluble metal salts are mainly found in the minerals of bone but other insoluble calcium salts such as calcium oxalate do occur. As with the first group, it is also possible to have contamination with metal salts. The metals may even be introduced by the processing. Rust in tap water is not unknown and may contaminate tissues during a washing step in the preparation.

Organically bound metals and their unmasking

The final group, where the minerals are bound into organic form, is the most important group and includes the iron in haemoglobin and the cytochromes.

There are several methods available for releasing such organically bound metals. Minerals need to be soluble and ionic before they can demonstrated since it is only the ions that react. Many of the difficulties with the techniques are related to this releasing or unmasking of the minerals without losing or relocating them. Releasing the minerals can sometimes be done by chemical treatments such as acid hydrolysis with hydrochloric acid or oxidation by hydrogen peroxide. If these can be shown to release all the metal then they are certainly the simplest solution.

Micro-incineration can unmask many metals

As an alternative to chemical unmasking the release of the metals can be achieved by burning off all the organic matter using **micro-incineration**. This changes all the organic minerals into salts and so the total content of metal can be seen. Incineration is done in a laboratory furnace at 500–600°C. Glass slides cannot withstand this high temperature so sections need to be mounted on quartz slides. For the best results oxygen needs to be excluded whilst the temperature is low ($< 500°C$) and only after this is air admitted. Oxidation then occurs rapidly and completely. The exclusion of air helps to remove the organic matter by preventing incomplete combustion products forming which then resist further oxidation. The slide is then carefully removed and cooled. The pattern of ash is quite extensive and usually the main tissue structures can be seen in outline. The pattern of ash is sometimes known by the somewhat grand name of a **spodogram**. It is very fragile and must be protected with a coverslip and then ringed. An alternative is to coat it by gently dipping it into a solution of celloidin. The celloidin then hardens and protects it but still allows reagents to penetrate and react with the released salts.

Micro-incineration with a Bunsen burner

Micro-incineration can also be more crudely done with a standard Bunsen burner. The tissue section on an ordinary slide is placed on an asbestos mat. A Bunsen burner is then picked up and the hot blue spot of the flame is played over the section so that the section passes through the bright blue edge of the flame where it is hottest. The section will turn brown initially and then turn from brown to white as the organic material burns off. There is no need to dewax paraffin sections as the wax will also burn off. Once the section has turned white it consists of only the mineral salts. The slide should then be covered to slow down cooling, as the slide is likely to shatter if cooling is rapid. The final ash can then be protected as before.

Micro-incineration is very rarely done. It is not suitable for all minerals, mercury will evaporate for example. It is a simple way to distinguish pure carbon deposits from silica as carbon will be burnt off in the process but silica will remain. It is also very difficult to precisely locate minerals within the tissue since by the time you have incinerated the section there is no tissue left and accurate location is not possible.

Spot test sensitivity and contamination

One further problem with mineral identification is contamination during preparation of the sections. Many of the histochemical spot tests are so sensitive that they will pick up contamination at very low concentrations. For the best and most reliable results ALL reagents should be completely free of the ions that are going to be demonstrated. This can be surprisingly difficult since some reagents will pick up ions very easily. Copper contamination from wax baths is not unknown and sections can be contaminated from metal forceps, scalpels and even microtome knives. Contamination should always be considered if results seem at all unexpected. If the wax block is prepared before you know that a histochemical test for mineral is needed then it may be too late and contamination may have already occurred. The opposite problem is the loss of minute deposits during processing, especially in acidic reagents. More materials are soluble at acid pH than in alkaline solutions but ideally neutral pH should be used.

In the following section a few of the more important minerals will be considered.

Calcium

Calcium deposits in the body come in a few main forms. Hydroxyapatite is the main mineral in teeth and bone. The mineralization in bone is critical for health while for some diseases the measurement of calcification is an important diagnostic aid. Strictly the calcification should be called mineralization as it includes metals other than calcium.

Von Kossa is useful for calcification but not specific for calcium

The von Kossa technique using silver to demonstrate mineralization has been explained already in the section on silver techniques and although important von Kossa is not really a method for calcium itself. Other forms of calcium often do not react with von Kossa, for example crystalline calcium carbonate and the calcified materials in invertebrates, so it is best regarded as a measure of bone mineral not a method for calcium.

Some dyes will complex with calcium

Some dyes can bind selectively to calcium and are more specific methods for calcium than the von Kossa method and they are also equally good at determining mineralization. Simple haematoxylin staining as with haematoxylin and eosin gives a distinctive blue colour with mineralized bone compared to the pink colour of osteoid. This is seen even better with an unmordanted haematoxylin when only the calcified material will stain. Alizarin red sulphonate (alizarin red S) is probably the most used of the simple dyes. Alizarin is not absolutely specific for calcium but also reacts with aluminium, barium and strontium. Aluminium and barium, however, give a slightly different colour and strontium is usually mixed with the calcium and is indistinguishable from it.

Alizarin can show bone development in embryos

One use for alizarin is in the Dawson technique for examining bones in embryos. This is a method of treating whole embryos so that the bony structures can be seen through the body tissues. The soft tissues of the embryo are macerated by treating them with strong hydroxide. This renders them softer and less likely to take up the stain. The bones are stained with alizarin and then the soft tissues are made transparent by soaking in glycerol which has a high refractive index and, like the organic clearing agents, makes soft tissues almost transparent. The stained bones can then be seen clearly through the translucent soft tissues.

Diseases in which calcium is deficient include rickets and osteomalacia which are caused by lack of vitamin D. Although dietary deficiency is now quite rare in this country as vitamin D is added to many foodstuffs, the diseases can still occur due to malabsorption in Crohn's disease.

Vitamin D can be synthesized in the skin by the action of UV light but the darker skins of some races prevent this formation of vitamin D in the skin. There is an occasional case of vitamin D deficiency in some Asian communities. Some chappatti flours also inhibit the absorption of calcium and this exaggerates the disease. Bone biopsies may be used to confirm the diagnosis.

Osteoporosis is a very important disease in post-menopausal women and causes skeletal deformities, bone pain and fractures. In the years immediately following the menopause bone mass may reduce by as much as 3% per year. Osteoporosis is usually diagnosed from the radiographic appearance rather than bone biopsy.

Drug and dye incorporation into bone during normal bone growth

Xylenol orange is another dye which can be incorporated into bone but is usually used as a vital stain when it is incorporated into new bone as it mineralizes. This is a useful way of locating where new bone is being formed but it is of course limited to animal studies. An alternative to the xylenol orange dye is the use of tetracycline antibiotics. These work in the same way and fluoresce quite strongly when bound to calcium in bone. The different tetracyclines fluoresce in different colours so, depending on the tetracyclines that have been used, it is possible to identify when particular parts of calcified structures formed. This can be useful even in humans since tetracyclines are used as antibiotics for the treatment of infections so some samples may include tetracyclines from their clinical use. This technique can employ a pulsed delivery with a short dose given to label newly formed bone and then a gap before a second dose. The sharp doses rapidly localize in the newly forming bone as discrete lines and the distance between them represents the rate of bone growth in the period between the two pulses. I have even seen the same effect in the tooth of a child who had been given three courses of tetracycline, where the tooth showed distinct lines corresponding to the growth between tetracycline treatments.

Magnesium

Magnesium is often found along with calcium in mineralized tissues but it can be identified as an independent ion by chelation with dyes. The dyes are thiazol yellow G and 4-(p-nitrophenylazo)-resorcinol (Magneson). The thiazol yellow gives a red colour to magnesium deposits while Magneson gives a blue colour.

Iron

Iron occurs in haemoglobin, myoglobin, cytochromes, ferritin and haemosiderin, in all of which it is organically bound. Iron is constantly recycled by the body with only small amounts being lost or gained under normal circumstances. Iron is poorly absorbed from the diet, particularly from vegetable sources, and women can become iron deficient due to the monthly losses of iron in the menstrual blood flow. Many women are prescribed iron tablets to supplement their dietary sources. If large amounts are absorbed then it can prove toxic and iron poisoning is a problem with children taking their parents' iron pills. This toxicity may be due to the iron generating free radicals which then damage the tissue.

Haemochromatosis is caused by excessive iron uptake

In the disease of primary haemochromatosis there is an excessive absorption of iron and the iron deposits as haemosiderin in many

Iron poisoning is one of the commonest causes of poisoning in children. In the USA there were 110,000 cases between 1986 and 1992 of whom 33 died. The immediate effects of iron overdose are to cause vomiting, diarrhoea and gastrointestinal bleeding. If the child recovers from these problems then there may be liver damage, heart failure and coma within 1–2 days. If the child survives and recovers from the initial toxicity then there may still be problems including liver damage up to 6 weeks later.

So the steps involved in producing a fluorescently labelled antibody are:

1. Prepare a pure antibody solution against a known antigen (e.g. anti-actin is prepared by injecting purified actin into an animal).
2. Treat the purified antibody with FITC to conjugate the dye and label the antibody.
3. Wash the labelled antibody solution free of unused FITC. This can be done by dialysis or gel filtration.

Labelled antibody will react with its specific antigen in the tissues

This labelled antibody can then be used at a suitable dilution to stain sections. Careful washing is needed but the technique is quite simple. The section can then be viewed with a fluorescent microscope, when any bound antibody will fluoresce showing the sites of antibody binding and this in turn identifies the sites of the antigen. Using the example of actin, the binding sites for anti-actin antibody would indicate the location of actin. This simple technique, involving just one antibody conjugated with FITC, is called the **direct immunofluorescent technique**.

Anti-nuclear antibodies occur in rheumatoid arthritis

In some diseases (e.g. rheumatoid disease) the patients produce an abnormal antibody that reacts with nuclear material. This anti-nuclear antibody is important for the diagnosis and prognosis of such diseases. The antibody is present in the patient's serum and can be identified using tissue sections or cell smears and staining using immunofluorescent methods. The anti-nuclear antibody will react with the nuclear proteins of several species and is not limited to human nuclei. Frozen sections of rat tissue can be used as test sections to detect if there is any antibody present in the patient's serum.

Human antibodies will be antigenic in other animals

Detection of immunoglobulin requires an antibody directed against immunoglobulin. This is an antibody against an antibody. This production of antibodies against antibodies is a little difficult to understand and follow the first time you come across it but it is a very useful technique. Human antibodies are proteins and can therefore act as antigens in a species other than humans. If an animal is injected with human antibody, then it produces, as usual, an antibody that will bind with its specific antigen which in this case is human antibody. Antibodies are immunoglobulins so the reagent is called anti-human immunoglobulin; if the animal it was

Anti-nuclear antibodies are found in a variety of disorders including rheumatoid disease, lupus erythematosis, mixed connective tissue disease and some liver disease. The antibodies are classed as autoimmune antibodies since they will react with antigens present in the patient. Autoimmune diseases can be diagnosed by detecting the free antibody in the patient's blood or by detecting bound antibody on the patients' cells.

Other autoimmune antibodies are also found and many seem to react with endocrine tissues but the significance of this is not known.

In some cases auto-immune antibodies are directed against a single organ (e.g. Hashimoto's thyroiditis) or against a whole number of different organs (e.g. systemic lupus erythematosis). The damage to the tissues may be caused directly by antibody or cellular immunity but can also occur by the production of immune complexes in the tissues. An immune complex is a combination of antibody and antigen which can become deposited in delicate tissues such as the kidney and the precipitated complex then causes the damage.

The terminology of antibodies often hinders understanding. The terms antibody and antigen are fairly well defined. An antigen is a foreign material which when introduced into the body stimulates the production of an antibody. The terminology for naming antibodies is to prefix their antigen with anti-. So anti-actin is an antibody against actin. In some cases (as in the accompanying text) it is important to know the animal in which the antibody was prepared. So, if an anti-actin was prepared in a rabbit it is termed rabbit anti-actin. If the antibody is prepared against an immunoglobulin (i.e. anti-antibody) then two species are needed – the one in which the antibody was made and the species from which the antigen (an Ig) came. Injecting rabbit immunoglobulin into a goat will produce goat anti-rabbit Ig. The first species is the species used to make the reagent and the second is the species of the antigen (in this case rabbit Ig).

The term serum is also in common use and can also cause confusion. Serum is the protein-rich fluid left after plasma has been allowed to clot and the clot has been removed. Serum contains all the antibodies but has lost the ability to clot. Serum has been the traditional material for immunology and the subject is often referred to as **serology** from this widespread use of serum. Unfortunately, a serum containing antibodies is referred to as an **antiserum**. This does not mean that it necessarily has antibodies against serum, just that it contains antibodies. The term antiserum is also loosely applied to monoclonal antibodies which are not even serum but antibody solutions from cell culture media.

prepared in was a rabbit it would be called rabbit anti-human immunoglobulin.

Human antibodies can be detected using anti-immunoglobulins

To detect if there is any anti-nuclear antibody in a patient's serum the following steps are needed:

1. The first step is to apply the patient's serum to frozen sections. If there is any anti-nuclear antibody present then it will bind to the nuclei.
2. The patient's serum is then washed away.
3. The section is then treated with FITC-conjugated anti-human immunoglobulin. The anti-human antibody will only bind to human antibody. In a rat section the only way that human antibody could be present would be if there was anti-nuclear antibody in the test serum which had bound to the rat nuclei.
4. Finally it is necessary to wash away the FITC-labelled antibody and examine the section for fluorescence. If the nuclei fluoresce then the patient's serum contained anti-nuclear antibodies.

The strength of the antibody can be measured

The immunofluorescent technique can be used to estimate the strength of the antibody by preparing a series of dilutions of the patient's serum and testing them for binding. The dilution that just gives a detectable positive reaction is taken as the **titre** of the serum. A serum that has a titre of 1/512 means that if the serum is diluted to 1 part of serum in 511 parts of buffer it will still give a detectable reaction, but if diluted to 1/1024 (twice as dilute) then no reaction can be detected.

Direct and indirect techniques

The anti-nuclear antibody technique uses two antibodies, the first or primary antibody is in the patient's serum and the second is prepared as an anti-antibody (Figure 10.1). Only the second antibody is conjugated. This **indirect technique** can be used to detect any antibody not just anti-nuclear antibodies in disease states. When a primary antibody is prepared by immunizing an animal there is no need to conjugate this primary antibody. Instead a second antibody is prepared in a different species against the immunoglobulins of the first species and this secondary antibody is conjugated with FITC.

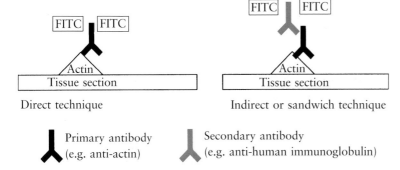

Figure 10.1 *Diagram of the direct and indirect antibody tehniques*

Indirect techniques can be used for any antigen

The idea of an indirect technique is perhaps easier to understand if the individual species are named. Anti-actin antibody can be prepared from a rabbit by immunizing it with pure actin. This antibody is not conjugated with fluorescein. Anti-rabbit antibody can be prepared by immunizing a goat with purified rabbit antibody. This is called **goat anti-rabbit immunoglobulin**. The antibody used to immunize the goat does not need to be the specific anti-actin antibody, any rabbit antibody will produce the same effect. The goat anti-rabbit antibody will react with any antibody from any rabbit. This antibody is conjugated and will be a general reagent for any rabbit antibody. So if we need to identify keratin then all that is needed is to prepare a new first antibody. This would mean raising in a rabbit some anti-keratin antibody and this will also be detected by the same goat anti-rabbit immunoglobulin that was used with the anti-actin antibody.

The indirect technique has many advantages

The indirect technique is a better method than the direct technique for the following reasons:

- As just explained it is not necessary to conjugate every antibody. This makes it cheaper since conjugation adds to the cost of an antibody.

- It is more sensitive since there can be more than one conjugated antibody bound to a single antigen site. In the direct technique only one conjugated antibody can be bound to an antigen site. In the indirect technique, although there can still only be one primary antibody bound to the antigen site, there can be several secondary antibodies bound to the primary antibody. Each of the secondary antibodies will have fluorescein attached to it. This increases the intensity of the fluorescence so smaller amounts of antigen can be detected.

- The increased sensitivity means that the antibodies can be used in a more dilute solution and this means that the reagents will be

Fluorescein labelling is the most frequent method of fluorescently labelling antibodies but there are other fluorescent dyes that have been used. Rhodamine and Texas red both have a red fluorescence and can be used as a second label when two different antigens are to be demonstrated in the same preparation. This double staining is useful for seeing how two materials are distributed and the relationship between them. The plant pigment phycoerythrin has also been used as it has a high fluorescent capability.

Besides labelling through the isothiocyanate derivatives it is also possible to use succinimidyl esters and sulphonyl halides as reactive forms of the dyes, and these will also react with the amine groups. These forms are more stable but are more difficult to produce and are less often used.

able to treat more sections. This reduces the cost of preparing a large number of slides.

Fluorescent labelling has some disadvantages

Fluorescent labelling is widely used not only in histology but also in microbiology and haematology. Immunofluorescence has several disadvantages for staining sections. The main disadvantages are:

- Observing fluorescence requires a special fluorescence microscope with a high power lamp and this is usually significantly more expensive than a simple microscope using visible light. This expense involves both in the initial equipment costs and the cost of replacement lamps.

- Fluorescence is always quite dim and observing the faint glow requires a darkened room and the observer needs to allow his eyes to become dark-adjusted before looking at the slides.

- It is difficult to counterstain the section with a dye since any fluorescence of the background might mask a dim positive reaction. In the absence of a counterstain it is therefore more difficult to accurately locate the position of the fluorescent material in relation to other structures.

- The fluorescence is not permanent. The dye will show fading or bleaching in a few days and will fade more quickly if it is examined under the microscope. Fading in microscope illumination can be sufficiently fast for it to be lost in minutes.

- It is difficult to photograph the fluorescence. The image is dim so a long exposure would be needed but the dye fades during long exposures.

Immunohistochemistry

The problems with fluorescein labels led to a search for other antibody labels including enzymes. The use of these histochemical labels is termed immunohistochemistry. Immuno-histochemistry uses enzymes to label the antibodies and histochemical tests to identify the sites of binding.

As was explained in a previous chapter, enzymes can be demonstrated in tissues and can give highly coloured, insoluble reaction products. An enzyme can also produce large amounts of coloured product if the incubation with the substrate is long enough. This allows visualization of very small amounts of enzyme and makes enzymes a prime labelling material providing some way can be found to link the enzyme and the antibody together. Although there are many enzymes that could be used the ones that have proved most popular are horse-radish peroxidase (HRP) and alkaline phosphatase (AP).

Initially chemicals were used to link the enzyme to the antibody

Having chosen an enzyme the next step is to link the enzyme and the antibody together. One of the first techniques used glutaraldehyde which is a bifunctional aldehyde. One aldehyde group can react with the protein of the antibody while the other reacts with the protein of the enzyme:

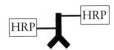

Thus glutaraldehyde crosslinks the antibody and enzyme in the same way that it crosslinks tissue proteins when it is used as a fixative. This technique worked quite well but there was a lot of wasted antibody since simply mixing the glutaraldehyde with a mixture of antibody and enzyme can result in a variety of combinations (Figure 10.2):

- The antibody can be crosslinked to another antibody. This combination could bind to the antigen but would not be able to be visualized since there is no enzyme present.
- The enzyme could be crosslinked to another enzyme. This combination could not bind to the antigen.
- Larger aggregations of several crosslinked proteins could form. These would either precipitate out of solution or would be simply too large to be able to approach the antigenic site and would not bind because of steric hindrance.
- Finally there would be a mixture of an antibody linked to an enzyme in small enough aggregations to be useful. This final group is the only type of reactant that could be used. The previous three types of combined proteins were not wanted and had to be removed from the solution.

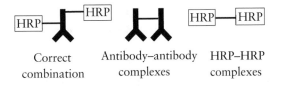

Correct   Antibody–antibody   HRP–HRP
combination   complexes   complexes

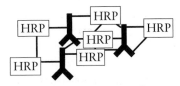

Large insoluble complexes

Figure 10.2 *Unwanted reactions between enzymes, glutaraldehyde and HRP*

The various forms could be effectively separated using gel filtration techniques so the antibody could be prepared as a pure form. It was simply very wasteful of reagent since significant amounts of the antibody were being discarded and lost.

The purified antibody–enzyme combination could be used by either the direct or sandwich method, the same as for fluorescein labelling. In this case indirect techniques are even more favoured since the labelling technique is so wasteful.

The major steps in the indirect enzyme-labelled antibody method using horse-radish peroxidase are:

1. Apply the primary antiserum to the sections. If there is any antigen present then the antibody will bind to it.
2. The primary antiserum is then washed away.
3. The section is then treated with enzyme-linked anti-immunoglobulin. This will bind to any primary antibody held in the section.
4. Wash away the excess labelled antibody.
5. Treat the section with the appropriate enzyme demonstration technique to develop the final colour. For horse-radish peroxidase this could be a mixture of hydrogen peroxide and diaminobenzidene in buffer.
6. Counterstain the tissue to show the general structure.

Sites of the enzyme will show as deposits of brown chromogen and these sites will be the position of the antigen.

Unlabelled antibody techniques

Since both the enzyme (e.g. HRP) and the antibody are proteins they can both act as antigens. It was realized that it was possible to link these components together by using a third antibody. This requires two different species of animal and three antibodies. The three antibodies needed are:

1. the primary antibody against the antigen prepared in a stated species (e.g. rabbit anti-actin);
2. an anti-horse-radish peroxidase antibody prepared in the same species (e.g. rabbit anti-HRP);
3. a bridging antibody against the immunoglobulin of the species used to prepare 1 and 2 (e.g. goat anti-rabbit Ig).

These are applied in sequence to the section (Figure 10.3).

The primary antibody (rabbit anti-actin) is applied first and binds to the antigen. After washing away the excess antibody the goat anti-rabbit immunoglobulin is applied and will bind to the rabbit anti-actin antibody. Since there is a large amount of the goat anti-rabbit immunoglobulin the binding will only use one of the binding sites available on the secondary antibody. When the final rabbit

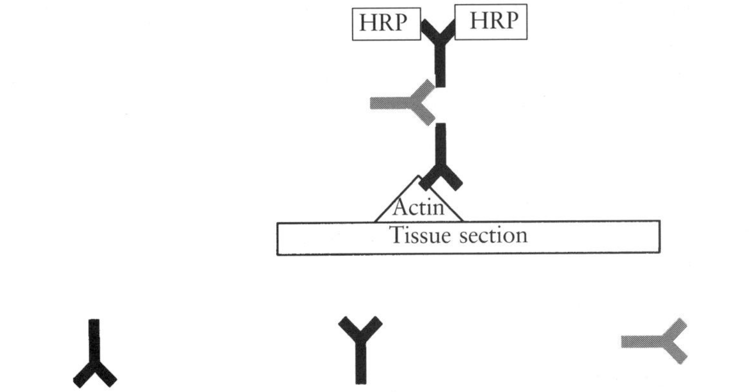

Figure 10.3 *Diagram of the unlabelled antibody method*

anti-HRP antibody is applied it will be trapped by the unused binding sites of the secondary antibody. The secondary antibody thus binds the primary antibody and the tertiary antibody by acting as a bridge between them.

The next step would be to add horse-radish peroxidase which would be trapped by the anti-HRP antibody. The enzyme can then be demonstrated as before and a brown chromogen deposit will indicate the sites of actin within the tissues.

The peroxidase–anti-peroxidase technique

Variations on this technique are now among the most popular techniques of immunohistochemistry. The horse-radish peroxidase enzyme and the anti-HRP antibody can be made as a single ready-prepared complex (peroxidase–anti-peroxidase or PAP) rather than having to add the final antibody and the enzyme as separate steps. The PAP complex consists of two antibodies and three peroxidase molecules in an almost cyclical structure. The complex is soluble and even though the enzyme is bound by the antibody its activity is not inhibited.

The PAP reagent can be easily purified

The PAP complex has another advantage. Since the PAP complex is prepared separately it can be purified more easily and this gives greater sensitivity and less background staining. The anti-peroxidase antibody needs to be very pure. If it is prepared in an animal then it is likely to be contaminated with non-specific antibodies. These antibodies will compete with the anti-peroxidase antibody for binding on to the bridging antibody and this will reduce the final colour. It is almost impossible to separate the specific and non-

With the unlabelled antibody technique it is also possible to repeat the processes involving the anti-HRP and HRP. By adding extra anti-HRP after the HRP has been added then the anti-HRP will bind to the HRP. By using a lot of anti-HRP it is possible to ensure that only one of the two binding sites is used. The other binding site can now bind more HRP. So by alternating the anti-HRP and HRP solutions the amount of HRP can be greatly increased. In practice the process is limited since there is also an increase in the background staining.

specific antibodies while they exist as individual molecules but the PAP complex is easier to purify.

If an impure serum from a rabbit immunized with peroxidase is mixed with peroxidase it will form the complex. The complex is now much larger than the other antibodies and can be separated by gel filtration to give a much purer preparation. The same technique can be used with alkaline phosphatase and is referred to as the APAAP (alkaline phosphatase–anti-alkaline phosphatase) method. The PAP and APAAP techniques have virtually completely replaced the simple unlabelled bridge technique from which they were originally developed.

The PAP technique is very sensitive but is longer and more complex than the simple direct immunofluorescence technique.

Endogenous enzymes may cause background reactions

One possible disadvantage of using enzymes as labelling reagents is that the tissue may contain similar enzymes. Alkaline phosphatases and peroxidases are common in tissues. The enzymes within the tissue are **endogenous** and if they are allowed to react with the substrate then they will produce the same chromogen as the exogenous enzyme used to label the antibody.

The presence of endogenous enzyme can be seen if a section is treated with the same technique as the test section but omitting the enzyme-labelled antibody step. Any colour produced can only be due to the tissue enzymes. This background is a nuisance and needs to be suppressed. One method is to inactivate the endogenous enzyme before performing the immunocytochemistry reaction and this is probably the best way if it can be done conveniently.

Blocking may be specific for the enzyme, e.g. using methanol containing 0.3% hydrogen peroxide will inhibit peroxidase enzymes. Alternatively the enzyme may be blocked non-specifically, e.g. using formaldehyde or other fixatives. This works quite well for the APAAP method and, since the technique is often carried out on paraffin wax processed tissue there is no need to deliberately inactivate the enzyme. The peroxidases in tissues are less easily inactivated in this way and even paraffin wax processed tissue may still retain significant peroxidase activity and may need to be specifically inactivated by using methanol/H_2O_2.

Antibodies may be absorbed non-specifically on to the tissues

The high sensitivity of the PAP method may itself cause difficulties if the bridging antibody is absorbed or adsorbed on to the tissue at sites where there is no antigen. The bridging antibody will then bind the PAP complex and give a non-specific background colour. This non-specific background can be eliminated by treating the section with a normal serum from the same species as the bridging antibody. So if the bridging antibody was goat anti-rabbit immunoglobulin then the section is first treated with diluted normal goat serum. Any binding sites capable of non-specific reaction with goat serum will absorb the non-immune serum and be blocked. The immune serum will not be absorbed and as a result the background will be cleaner.

The PAP technique is not reliably quantitative

Enzyme labelling techniques and particularly the bridging techniques are not quantitative. The method produces such high amplification that even small amounts of antigen can give strong results. If the antigen is very concentrated in the tissues then it may even give a weaker response.

High concentrations of antigen can block the absorption of the PAP

This incongruous result is due to the bridging antibody being effectively blocked by the high concentration of primary antibody that is bound when there is a lot of antigen in the tissue (Figure 10.4).

Following the previous example, the goat anti-rabbit IgG antibody is divalent and can bind two rabbit antibodies. Provided the rabbit antibodies are well separated within the tissues and there is a great excess of goat antibodies, then each goat anti-rabbit IgG molecule will only have one of its binding sites attached to the primary rabbit antiserum. The second binding site will then attach to the PAP complex. However, if there is a lot of antigen then the antibodies will be closer together and the concentration may be locally higher than the concentration of the goat anti-rabbit immunoglobulin. This results in many or indeed most of the bridging antibodies binding with **both** of its binding sites to the primary antiserum. There will be few or no free binding sites for trapping the PAP so the final colour will be less. This mechanism also explains why using a more dilute reagent will give a stronger result when there is a lot of antigen in the specimen. The PAP technique should therefore be used to detect the presence of antigen but not used to attempt to quantify the amount, even approximately.

Controls are needed to ensure specificity and correct technique

To ensure the technique is working correctly a minimum of three controls are needed. These must be done at the same time and in the same way as the test section:

1. Known positive control (weakly reacting is best). This control

The PAP and APAAP methods are better for most purposes in histology but fluorescent methods still have their advantages. The fluorescence can be easier to locate if there is not a great deal of antigen present; for example trying to locate a few bacteria in a large section. Secondly, the method can be quantitative by measuring the fluorescence. Finally, the fluorescence shows where the antibody is located and can move with the antibody. Enzyme labelling only shows where the antibody is if the antibody does not move. If the antibody can move then it will show where the antibody was at the time the chromogen was being produced. This can be important in some applications. For example the membrane of a cell is constantly being recycled and the recycling can be demonstrated by 'capping'. An antibody against a cell-membrane protein is applied to living cells. The membrane will be evenly labelled all around the membrane. As the membrane is recycled by being drawn into the cell the membrane proteins form a cap just above where the membrane is being drawn back into the cytoplasm.

Initially even labelling   'Capping' of the label

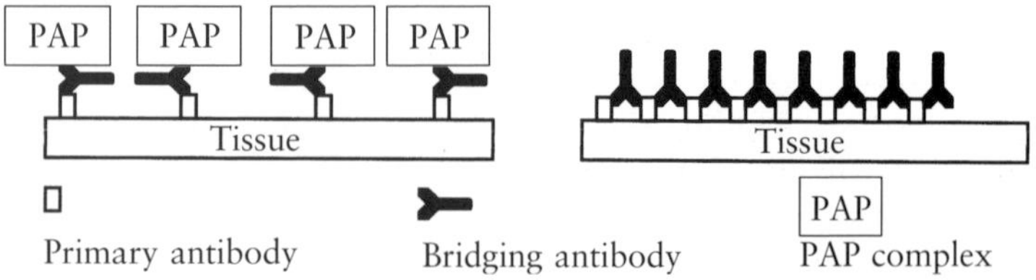

Figure 10.4 *Effect of high antigen density on staining. On the left the primary antibodies are widely spaced and so the bridging antibody is not saturated and has free binding sites to bind the PAP complex. On the right the primary antibodies are close enough to allow the antibody to use both binding sites in binding to the primary antibody. There are no free binding sites for the PAP complex*

must show a positive reaction. A negative shows a failure to react and so a negative result in the test section is unreliable.

2. Known negative control. This should be negative. Any positive result shows if there is a non-specific result. Any positive reactions in the test section would be unreliable.

3. A control using the test section but omitting the first (primary) antibody. This control should be negative. If this is positive it may indicate an endogenous enzyme in the test section, or non-specific absorption of one of the other reagents.

The above three controls should detect any discrepancies. If any unexpected results are seen then they can be further investigated by using extra control steps to determine the nature of the discrepancy (e.g. blocking controls, no application of any antibody, pretreatment with HRP).

Avidin–biotin methods

Avidin is a glycoprotein found in egg white that binds strongly to the vitamin biotin. This binding is much stronger than the usual antibody binding and is very difficult to disrupt. By linking biotin to the antibody a complex can be formed that is very stable.

Avidin was originally discovered when rats that were fed a diet rich in raw egg whites began to suffer from biotin deficiency. The avidin was holding the biotin so effectively in the rat gut that the animals became deficient. The investigation of this toxicity of egg protein led to the discovery of avidin. It is unlikely that eggs will have the same effect in humans as the eggs are usually cooked and the number of eggs that are eaten is usually quite small. Biotin is produced in quite large quantities by the normal gut bacteria and deficiency in humans is extremely rare.

Proteins can be labelled with biotin

Biotin can be conjugated to most proteins, carbohydrates and nucleic acids by using an active derivative. For proteins this is usually sulpho-*N*-succinimidobiotin which can add the biotin on to free amino groups. The biotin is a small molecule and does not usually interfere with the activity of the protein. Biotinylation of antibodies is therefore an alternative method of labelling.

Avidin is used to bind on to the biotinylated protein

The biotin is then detected by using avidin that binds to the biotin (Figure 10.5). The avidin itself has a label attached which can be fluorescent or an enzyme. The most popular of these techniques uses an avidin–biotin complex ('ABC') which combines several avidin molecules and several peroxidase molecules. The enzymes

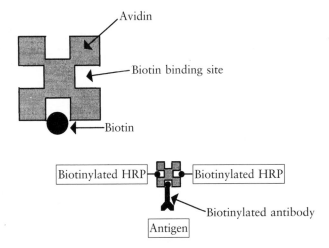

Figure 10.5 *Avidin–biotin method. The avidin acts as a bridge between the biotinylated antibody and the biotinylated horse-radish peroxidase. The avidin in the lower diagram shows a free biotin binding site which can be used to bind the 'ABC' reagent*

are biotinylated so that they will bind to the avidin molecule. This complex is much larger than the PAP complex and contains more peroxidase, but despite this the ABC method is about comparable in sensitivity to the PAP method.

The ratio of biotin and avidin can be varied

There is a more biotin-rich complex colloquially known as 'CBA' that can be used to boost the activity. The CBA is used after the ABC reagent and is bound to the ABC complex by its extra biotin and so adds an extra layer. The CBA can then be followed by an extra treatment with the ABC reagent which can bind to the excess biotin in the CBA. This in turn can be followed by ABC and so on. This alternation of biotin-rich and avidin-rich layers could be compounded to give any number of repeats, but this is pointless as beyond two or three extra steps the added sensitivity will be counterbalanced by a loss of specificity.

The avidin in all the above techniques can be replaced by the protein **streptavidin** which is extracted from a streptomyces organism and has similar binding properties and is preferred by many workers because it gives less background staining.

The use of biotin as a label also has its own problems since many tissues, including liver and kidney, have significant amounts of endogenous biotin and can give false positive results.

Immunogold labelling

Immunogold labelling uses particles of colloidal gold to label the antibody. The colloidal gold will adsorb on to the protein and act as a visible label. This is very popular with electron microscopists as the spherical gold particles are easily seen in the EM. The colloidal gold can be made in differing particle sizes so that it is possible to use two different sized labels to identify two antigens in the same preparation. Although mainly used for EM colloidal gold can be made visible for light microscopy by using silver solutions. The silver reagents react with the gold and produce an enhanced blackening easily seen by light microscopy.

Antigen retrieval methods

The fluorescent antibody technique usually only works well on fresh frozen tissue but the high sensitivity of the PAP and ABC methods allows them to be used on paraffin embedded sections. This has probably been one of their major advantages since the methods can be applied to routine blocks with no need to plan in advance for the use of immunostaining, and old blocks from the archives can be used quite effectively. Indeed it is even possible to perform the techniques on stained sections from which the cover-slips have been removed. The results from paraffin sections can, however, sometimes be disappointing since the fixation and processing can alter the antigens. To restore the full immunoreactivity of the sections various techniques have been tried. These techniques are referred to as unmasking of the antigen or **antigen retrieval methods**.

Enzyme retrieval

The first method involved the use of enzymes to digest away some of the protein to expose the masked antigenic sites. Usually it is a proteolytic enzyme, such as trypsin or pepsin, that is used to remove protein. The enzymes need to be freshly prepared as they lose activity once in solution. This works well in most instances but can be very sensitive to the conditions of incubation. Too long an incubation may remove excessive protein and associated antigen whilst too short an incubation may not fully unmask the antigen. The timing is also very dependent on fixation. This dependence is both for the type of fixative used, with formaldehyde generally being preferred, and also on the length of fixation, with long fixation needing longer digestion. Because of these variables it is usually necessary to test the timing and the technique for each batch of enzyme and sometimes for each individual specimen to get optimal staining.

This variability has led to some workers to question the validity of the technique and arguing that some of the results may represent an artefact of the digestion process rather than the site of preformed antigen. However, if well controlled, the technique does seem to give reliable and useful results and has been widely adopted for paraffin sections but is less useful for fresh tissue.

Heat retrieval

An alternative to using enzymes is to heat the section. Simple heating is insufficient and it requires prolonged exposure to boiling or superheated fluid to achieve the retrieval. Usually a sodium citrate solution buffered to a slightly acid pH is used, and the heating can be achieved by using a microwave oven or a pressure cooker.

Microwave retrieval. In the microwave method the dewaxed sections are placed in buffer in a microwave and heated at full power for 10–30 min depending on the antigen to be unmasked, the power of the microwave and the fixation of the tissue. The fluid rapidly boils and if this is being done in a Coplin jar, which holds about 50 ml of fluid, it results in boiling off of the fluid and often the buffer spills out so that the fluid needs to be constantly replenished. By using larger containers with an excess of buffer it may be possible to have sufficient fluid to avoid the need to replenish. The sections are allowed to cool in the buffer and then transferred to distilled water. This method is rapidly gaining popularity as it does not need to be optimized for different batches of enzyme.

Pressure cooker retrieval. Pressure cookers are an alternative way to heat the sections and use higher temperatures since water boils at a higher temperature at higher pressures. An ordinary stainless steel domestic pressure cooker is used and it is partially filled with citrate buffer and brought to the boil at normal pressure (the cooker is not sealed) before putting in the slides. The pressure cooker is then sealed and brought back to the boil at raised pressure. Most pressure cookers work at 1 atmosphere above normal pressure and this raises the boiling point of water to about 120°C. The increased temperatures reached mean that antigen retrieval times are much shorter, typically 2–4 min once the full pressure is reached. Pressure cookers can also treat many more slides at once than a microwave oven.

It is also possible to use two methods of retrieval by microwaving the sections first, cooling them to 37°C and then treating them with a protease.

The choice of retrieval method is largely determined by personal preference, the tissue preparation and the antigen being sought. Often there are several different techniques being employed within the same laboratory for different purposes. One beneficial aspect of the use of retrieval methods is that the antibodies can often be used in more dilute solutions with dilution factors in excess of 1/10,000 being cited in some papers.

> Dry heating of sections does not seem to unmask antigens in the same way as wet heat. It seems likely that there is a hydrolysis effect and the energy needed to activate this is quite high. Simple boiling of the section is less efficient. The microwaves probably produce temperatures above the normal boiling point within the solution and pressure cookers also have a higher temperature than the standard boiling point of water.

Lectins were originally identified by their ability to agglutinate red blood cells. The agglutination can be specific for certain blood groups since the blood group antigens are made of sugars and the different blood groups have different terminal sugars. Lectins can also be toxic in some cases, since if they are absorbed intact without being digested they will agglutinate the red cells in blood and cause a haemolytic disorder. Some types of bean contain sufficient lectin concentrations to cause disease in this way if they are eaten uncooked. Not all lectins are dangerous poisons and they are currently being investigated for possible use in drug delivery to specific sites.

Labelling of other proteins

Proteins other than antibodies can also be labelled using the same general methods as explained above.

Lectin histochemistry

Lectins are plant, or occasionally animal, proteins which bind to sugar molecules rather than antigens but otherwise the reaction has much in common with antibody binding. They are not immune proteins but occur endogenously in the tissues of the plant without needing to 'immunize' it. Like antibodies they can bind more than one sugar (they are polyvalent). Unlike antibodies many lectins need specific cations to bind effectively and these need to be added, e.g. Concanavalin A needs calcium ions to bind effectively. Lectins may be highly toxic since they can interfere with sugar interactions.

Only terminal sugars react

The sugars to which the lectins bind can be part of proteins (glycoproteins) or can be complex carbohydrates or in the form of mucins, but in all cases only the terminal sugars can be accessed. Sugars buried inside a protein or bound inside polysaccharides are not usually available to the lectins and will not be detected.

Lectins can be used as very precise reagents for locating sugars in tissues. Table 10.1 lists some lectins and their specificities. Lectins do sometimes react with other sugars but with a decreased binding strength. The use of lectins in histochemistry has greatly increased in the past few years as the importance of carbohydrates in cell recognition, cell adhesion and metabolic control has been realized.

Lectins can be located by several different methods

The lectins can be simply treated as an antigen and injected into an animal to raise antibodies against them and used in one of the labelling strategies already explained. Lectins can be applied to tissue sections and, after washing away the excess, any bound lectin can be identified by a standard immunotechnique. Lectins are also available as fluorescent conjugates, biotinylated lectins and

Table 10.1   *Examples of some lectins and their specificities*

Lectin	Abbreviation	Source	Specificity
Concanavalin A	Con A	*Canavalia ensiformis*	α-Mannose, α-glucose, GlcNAc
Wheatgerm agglutinin	WGA	*Triticum vulgare*	GlcNAc-β-1,4-GlcNAc
Horse gram lectin	DBA	*Dolichos biflorus*	GalNAc-α-1,3-GalNAc
Gorse lectin	UAE	*Ulex europaeus*	α-L-Fucose
Horseshoe crab lectin	LPA	*Limulus polyphemus*	N-Acetylneuraminic acid

enzyme-labelled lectins. These can be employed in a similar fashion to antibodies labelled in these ways.

Finally, lectins can occasionally be demonstrated using carbohydrate-containing enzymes. Glucose oxidase for example contains about 18% carbohydrate and the lectin can bind to the sugars present in the enzyme. The glucose oxidase can then be simply demonstrated using an enzyme technique. This greatly simplifies the technique compared to most other labelling methods. This works well for Concanavalin A but is less successful with other lectins as the specific sugars they bind to are not always available in the enzyme. Horse-radish peroxidase can also be used in the same way but suffers slightly from the presence of endogenous peroxidase, whilst human tissue does not contain any glucose oxidase activity so there is no background staining.

Protein A

Protein A is a staphylococcal protein that has a very specific affinity for the Fc part of mammalian IgG. It can be used in the same way as an anti-immunoglobulin. The protein A can be obtained commercially labelled with fluorescent dyes, biotin and enzymes. One benefit of using protein A is that it is not species specific and will detect most mammalian IgG. This is sometimes useful since it reduces the need to have several different anti-immunoglobulins when using primary antisera from different animal species. Its disadvantage is that it cannot be used in tissues containing endogenous IgG. Anti-human IgG can be used on rat lymph nodes as they will not contain human IgG, but protein A cannot be used on any lymph nodes as it will react with all mammalian IgG.

Specific receptors

Hormones will be bound by their specific receptors within the tissues and this can be used to detect the location of such receptors. This is fairly straightforward if the hormone is a protein and can be labelled in the same way as other proteins.

Some receptors can be detected by using exogenous proteins that will bind to the receptor. These techniques, using specific binding materials, are often unique and although useful and important do not have much in common beyond the fact that they bind tightly with a receptor within the tissue and that they can be labelled or conjugated by one of the methods already outlined without altering their binding ability. For example, α-bungarotoxin is found in the venom of a Taiwanese snake and binds to the acetylcholine receptor of the neuromuscular junction and this can be used to locate and identify the receptors. The α-bungarotoxin is available labelled with biotin and fluorescein. The general concept of labelling a protein that binds to the tissue in some specific way applies to all such exogenous binding materials. The source of the binding agent, however, can be quite varied.

There is one final labelling technique that can be applied to many materials and that is autoradiography which is the subject of the next chapter.

Suggested further reading

Brooks, S.A., Leatham, A.J.C. and Schumacher, U. (1997). *Lectin Histochemistry*. Oxford: BIOS/Royal Microscopical Society.

Carleton, S.J. (1996). Immunofluorescent techniques, in *Theory and Practice of Histological Techniques* (eds J.D. Bancroft and A. Stevens). Edinburgh: Churchill Livingstone.

Kiernan, J.A. (1990). *Histological and Histochemical Methods*. Oxford: Pergamon.

Self-assessment questions

1. Define the terms antibody and antigen and explain briefly why antibodies are useful as histochemical reagents.
2. Outline how fluorescein is used as an antibody labelling material.
3. What are the disadvantages of the immunofluorescent technique?
4. Name two enzymes that are used in immunological staining?
5. Outline the steps needed in the PAP (or APAAP) technique.
6. How can the PAP technique be used in EM?
7. What is meant by antigen retrieval and how can it be achieved?
8. Describe the use of lectins in histochemistry.
9. What is the main use of immunogold labelling?
10. What is the purpose of avidin in the ABC technique of antibody labelling?

Key Concepts and Facts

Antibodies

- Antibodies bind to a single specific antigen.

- Antibodies can be used in histology providing they are labelled to make them visible.

Immunofluorescence

- Fluorescein can be attached to antibodies to make them fluoresce.

- Antibodies can act as antigens so anti-antibodies can be prepared.

- Anti-antibodies are species specific.

- Rabbit anti-human Ig is an antibody prepared in a rabbit which has been injected with human antibody.

- The sandwich or indirect technique uses two antibodies. One is the primary antibody to detect the tissue antigen and the other is a secondary fluorescent antibody to detect bound primary antibody.

- Indirect immunofluorescence using two antibodies is usually more sensitive than direct immunofluorescence that uses only one labelled antibody.

Immunohistochemistry

- Immunohistochemistry uses an enzyme to label antibodies. The enzyme is demonstrated by a histochemical reaction and this locates the antibody bound to tissue antigen.

- Enzymes are proteins and can act as antigens and anti-enzyme antibodies will be produced.

- Unlabelled antibody techniques use three antibodies, none of which are chemically modified.

- Unlabelled antibody techniques are more sensitive than immunofluorescence.

- Antigen retrieval techniques use enzymes or heat to unmask antigen sites and allow antibodies to react with the antigen.

- Antigen retrieval techniques may sometimes give false results.

- Other commercial labelling systems are available.

- Other materials can be labelled in the same way as antibodies.

Chapter 11
Autoradiography

Learning objectives

After studying this chapter you should confidently be able to:

Outline the principle of autoradiography.

Name some radioisotopes commonly used in autoradiography and the nature of their radiations.

Describe the two types of emulsion used in autoradiography.

Outline the possible problems in autoradiography.

The first autoradigraph was done before there was any knowledge of radioactivity and even before radioactivity was even suspected. Autoradiography was the first method of identifying radioactivity. Uranium salts were thought to be fluorescent and Antoine Henri Becquerel was testing some salts and he left them on top of a paper-covered film in a draw ready to irradiate them with light the following day. They were left unused for a few days so rather than irradiating them he decided to just develop the film anyway. He was surprised to see blackening since fluorescence should not occur in the absence of light. This was the first indication of material producing unknown rays in the absence of heating or absorption of light.

Autoradiography is a method of accurately following the fate of chemicals in cells and organs using radioactive isotopes (radioisotopes) as labels. It is widely used to trace the routes of metabolism of drugs within animals and so this will be used as an example to show how an autoradiography investigation is planned and carried out, but the applications of autoradiography are very widespread and it is one of the most useful techniques in research.

The fate of a drug in the body involves two phenomena:

- firstly, how and where it is distributed within the body;
- secondly, how it is metabolized and excreted.

Ideally we would like to be able to follow both of these processes. The actual concentrations of most drugs within cells and tissues are generally quite low and so detecting the drug using conventional chemical tests would be difficult or impossible. To overcome this problem radioactive materials are used which can allow the detection of a few molecules of drug.

The process of autoradiography

The steps in autoradiography

The first step is to prepare some of the drug by replacing one of the normal stable isotopes with a radioactive isotope. The drug is then administered to an animal or put into a tissue culture medium. The drug is absorbed and distributed in the tissues and cells and may be metabolized. Sections of the animal tissues can be made. The

Figure 11.1 *Outline of the steps in autoradiography*

1. Prepare some radioactively labelled drug.

2. Administer to a laboratory animal.

3. Take tissue samples and prepare sections.

4. Cover the section with photographic emulsion.

5. Leave to allow radioactivity to affect the film, then develop the emulsion. Blackened areas show the sites of the radiolabelled material.

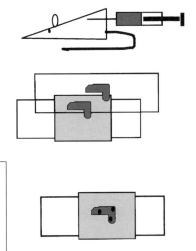

radioactive isotope will decay and emit radiation which can be detected using photographic film that reacts to the radiation in the same way as it would to light. The exposed film is developed in the same way as for photography and areas where there has been radioactivity will show as black areas (Figure 11.1). Only a few atoms decaying radioactively are needed to detect their position in the tissues so it is extremely sensitive. It is also necessary to be able to locate the film and the original section accurately so that the position of the isotope can be determined.

Autoradiography can also detect metabolic products

Not only is the distribution of the drug identified but also the way in which it is modified by the cells. Metabolism of the drug can be followed by autoradiography since, as the compound is broken down or changed by the cells or enzymes, the radioactive atoms will be incorporated into the breakdown products. By sampling over a period of time the fate of the drug can be followed up to its final excretion from the body. Although the body is always full of thousands of different metabolites only the radioactive drug and its metabolites are actually traced. This is possible since all the non-labelled compounds are ignored because they lack radioactivity and so do not register on the autoradiogram. Although autoradiogra-

Some elements have no isotopes that can be used for autoradiography. There are, for example, no useful isotopes of oxygen, nitrogen or chlorine. So labelling cannot be done for every atom in the molecule and the fate of some atoms must be guessed. In some cases this can be determined by using non-radioactive isotopes and using mass spectrometry to determine their fate. This can be done with oxygen which has a heavy but non-radioactive isotope.

phy is relatively simple to do, it requires careful planning to give good results since there are many potential pitfalls in the technique.

Choice of label and site of labelling

Labelling involves making a sample of the drug with one or more radioactive atoms. This is done by synthesizing the drug starting from a radioactive precursor. Many standard synthetic reagents are available from commercial sources so it is possible to make almost any compound. It is not, however, simple or cheap and should be done by an expert chemist since the radioactivity is dangerous and the preparations are usually done on a very small scale since the radioactive starting compounds are so expensive.

It is important to think carefully about the label before getting the radiolabelled drug synthesized.

Choice of radioisotope

It is not possible to replace every individual element since not all atoms have suitable radioisotopes (see Box). Radioactive decay can produce three forms of radiation as described in Table 11.1.

α-Particles

The α-particles are quite large and heavy. They are able to penetrate only a short distance through tissues or photographic film so they always affect the film very close to the site of the decaying atom and the accuracy of localization is good when using α-particles. It is made even better since the α-particle causes many electrons to be displaced as it passes through the photographic film so that its track can be seen as a straight line. If the lines all converge on one point (Figure 11.2) then the position of the isotope can be very accurately located.

Table 11.1 *Properties of radioactive emissions*

Type of radiation	Nature	Charge	Applications
α	Helium nucleus	+	Good localization but few α-emitters are interesting biologically
β	Electron	−	Localization poorer than α-particles but many of the atoms found in biological specimens have β-emitting isotopes
γ	Electromagnetic radiation	0	Useless for autoradiography but can be a nuisance since γ-rays are often emitted along with β-particles

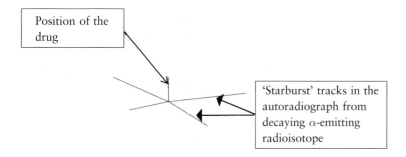

Position of the drug

'Starburst' tracks in the autoradiograph from decaying α-emitting radioisotope

Figure 11.2 *Appearance of the effect of α-decay in an autoradiogram. The centre point of the tracks indicates the location of α-emitting isotopes*

Unfortunately most of the α-emitting isotopes are not common elements in biological molecules so, although α-emitters would be good for autoradiography, they are rarely used in biology.

γ-Emitters

γ-Emitters are useless for autoradiography since γ-rays can travel very large distances from their origin. So even if they do cause blackening of the film it may be several millimetres away from their origin. Since γ-rays are emitted along with β-particles they can be a cause of background blackening of the film which is a nuisance.

β-particles are usually used in autoradiography

β-Particles are relatively light and have the same negative charge as the electrons in the outer shells of atoms. The β-particles are therefore often deflected by the electron shells of atoms. As a result of the deflections the electrons do not travel through the tissues or the autoradiographic film in straight lines but tend to wander around. Depending on their energy they may cause blackening some distance away from the isotope's actual position. They also do not leave tracks in the film since they dislodge comparatively few atoms from the radiographic emulsion.

If there are many radioactive disintegrations at the same point then there will be a lot of grains forming a 'cloud' around the sites of the radioactivity. The location of the isotope is somewhere within this cloud of dots but its exact position can only be an estimate (Figure 11.3).

β-Emitting isotopes include useful elements such as carbon, hydrogen and sulphur

There are, however, a lot of very useful β-emitters (Table 11.2). Suitable isotopes include hydrogen (tritium), carbon, sulphur and phosphorus. With β-rays the localization is affected by the energy of the radiation which is usually measured in electron volts (eV). Tritium (^{3}H) is one of the best isotopes for localization as it has a

Autoradiography is sometimes confused with microradiography. Microradiography involves placing a small piece of tissue or a tissue section on to a piece of film and then irradiating it with X-rays or γ-rays. This is similar to ordinary radiographic methods used in medicine to visualize bones and teeth and will detect radio-opaque materials in the section. Autoradiography is different in using radioactivity within the tissue and using mainly poorly penetrating β-particles, and it detects radiolabelled materials.

Figure 11.3 *The track of β-particles in an autoradiographic emulsion: (a) shows the path of the particle; (b) shows the sites of silver grains. Only one or two points on the β-particle's track leave a silver grain. With β-particles the accuracy of localization is less precise and all that can be assumed is that the radioactivity is somewhere within a circle*

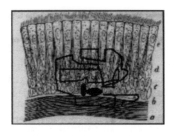

(a)

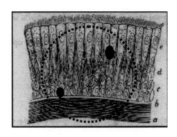

(b)

low energy emission. Tritium can even be used in the electron microscope to localize to the subcellular level, for example it can determine whether the drug is in the nucleus or the cytoplasm. With very careful technique it is even possible to estimate whether the isotope was in a mitochondrion or in the cytosol or, in the case of the nucleus, to which chromosome it was bound.

The effective resolution (see Table 11.2) indicates how accurately the position of the isotope can be determined. Carbon and sulphur are quite good for light microscopy magnifications and can certainly locate the isotope to individual cells. Phosphorus is less accurate for microscopy but is still useful for macroscopic and electrophoretic uses and can be relied upon to locate the material to small groups of cells.

The half-life of the isotope is important

As well as the energy of the β-particles from the isotope it is often important to consider the half-life of the isotope. The half-life is a measure of how quickly the atoms decay. Radioactive decay is a random event so it is only possible to be specific about the behaviour of many atoms and not individual atoms. We can never tell when an individual atom will decay but we can be quite accurate in saying that of a thousand atoms half will have decayed in a set time. That time is the half-life of the isotope. Half-lives vary tremendously. Carbon and tritium have long half-lives (5570 years and 12.3 years) but phosphorus is relatively short-lived (14 days). Isotopes with long half-lives are usually more convenient

Table 11.2   *Radioisotopes and their properties*

	Energy (keV)	*Half-life ($t_{\frac{1}{2}}$)*	*Effective resolution (μm)*
^{3}H (tritium)	19	12.4 years	0.5
^{14}C	156	5730 years	2–5
^{32}P	1710	14.3 days	5–10
^{35}S	167	87.4 days	2–5

experimentally as they can be used over long periods, so experiments can last several weeks without significant loss of radioactivity. With phosphorus the experiment needs to be quite brief. If the experiment required a 2-month time-scale then, by the end of the experiment, only about 6% of the original isotope would still be radioactive.

A second advantage of a long half-life is that the amount of blackening seen in the photographic emulsion can be increased by prolonging the time of exposure of the photographic film. Provided the radioactivity continues undiminished for a long time the radioactivity will continue to expose the film and increase the density of the image. With a short half-life such as using phosphorus, doubling the exposure will not increase the blackening effect very much. With an exposure time of 28 days (by no means unusual to detect very low concentrations of drug) three-quarters of all the radioactivity will have already occurred and leaving the specimen for the rest of eternity would only result in 25% more radioactive decay and 25% more blackening.

The safety also varies with half-life. Isotopes with long half-lives may cause disposal problems since they will remain radioactive long after the experiment has finished. An isotope with a short half-life will lose its radioactivity in simple storage and can be more easily discarded without worrying about the radiation hazard. Storing phosphorus for 1 year will make it non-radioactive.

Safety is important as isotopes may concentrate in the body

The other aspects of safety are concerned with concentration in the body. Tritium is often rapidly diluted in the body because of the large amount of hydrogen particularly in water but phosphorus concentrates in bone. This location does, however, also depend on the form of the isotope. If it is incorporated into a molecule it is not the nature of the isotope but the nature of the molecule that is important. Weaker radiations (e.g. tritium) do not penetrate far and are easily blocked even by air. Unless the isotopes actually get into the body they will not cause any damage since the dead cells on the skin will prevent the radiations reaching living cells. If they are ingested then the isotopes will come into direct contact with cells and are then dangerous.

My own choice would be tritium as it is long-lived, relatively safe and gives the best localization.

Which atoms in the drug are labelled is important

The site of labelling must be suitable. Ionizable or exchangeable atoms are of no use as they will not follow the compound. Many H atoms fall into this category but carbon is more often stable within the compound and will be a better labelling site. For example, take the case of acetic acid. If we were to label it with tritium it is vital

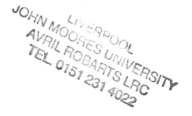

that we choose the right atom. If we synthesize the acetic acid so that the tritium is the acidic hydrogen in the carboxyl group then, when the acetic acid dissociates in water, the tritium will be lost into the fluid:

$$CH_3COOH + H_2O = CH_3COO^- + OH^- + 2H^+$$

It will not act as a tracer for the acetic acid. If, however, we synthesize the acetic acid with tritium attached as one of the hydrogens in the methyl group, then it will not be so easily displaced and can be used to follow the acetic acid.

Double labelling is possible in which two different atoms are replaced. For example, it would be possible to label the acetic acid with ^{14}C replacing the carbon in the carboxyl group and with tritium attached to the methyl carbon. If the acetic acid became split into the carboxyl group and the methyl group it would be possible to track both fragments separately.

Administration and metabolism of the labelled compound

Once the labelled drug has been synthesized it can then be administered. Usually this involves several small animals such as rats or mice being given the drug at the same time so that by examining animals at different times the fate of the drug can be followed. The drug can be given by mouth or injected, as appropriate to the drug being tested. The animals are then allowed to metabolize the drug for differing periods before being killed and prepared for histology.

How much of the labelled drug to give, how long to leave the animals and how frequently to sample the group of animals are all crucial questions but it is difficult to give any guidelines since the answers are unique to each experiment. In some cases it may be necessary to do a pilot study to get an idea of the right answers rather than being able to predict them theoretically.

Histological preparation

At the end of the experiment the fresh tissue obtained from the animal must be sectioned and the processing of the tissue needs to be considered carefully. The main need is to ensure that the material is not lost or redistributed by the processing. So questions need to be asked at every step in the process. Ideally these questions are all answered long before the experiment begins so that there is no delay in knowing how to treat the tissue once the animal is killed.

Fixation is an important choice

Questions that need to be considered include: 'Does the tissue need

Autoradiography can never be a diagnostic tool since it involves administering radioactivity to the subject and usually involves killing the subject to recover the tissues. The results of autoradiography can sometimes be confirmed in humans by using positron-emitting isotopes. The positrons can be detected using detectors outside the body and the fate of compounds can be followed. The positrons are detected using tomography equipment which locates the emission in three dimensions. These investigations are called PET scans (positron emission tomography).

Chapter 12
Exfoliative cytology and related techniques

Learning objectives

After studying this chapter you should confidently be able to:

Outline the advantages of exfoliative cytology.

Indicate why cytology can be used for screening.

Describe how a smear can be prepared and stained.

Describe the normal constituents of a smear.

Describe the changes that occur in gynaecological smears with age, menstrual cycle and pregnancy.

Outline the appearances of a smear showing inflammation and name the common causes of inflammation.

Describe the changes in smears in premalignant and malignant states.

Outline why a smear may be considered inadequate.

At first the idea of using shed cells for diagnosis was resisted since it seemed unreliable. Since only a sample of surface cells is examined it was thought that a small or deep tumour would be missed and the easy accessibility of the cervix for histological biopsy made cytology unnecessary. Cytological diagnosis also relies on different criteria to histological sections since the relationship between cells is lost. It was only the persistence of Dr George Papanicolaou that showed the potential of the method. It still took many years before it became fully accepted. Papanicolaou published his first paper on cancer diagnosis using smears in 1928 but it was not until after the Second World War that it became a recognized clinical method. Cervical screening in the UK began in the late 1940s with an early British pioneer in the field being Stanley Way in Gateshead who set up a screening service in 1948.

One of the major problems with histological diagnosis is the need for a piece of tissue to prepare sections. This means surgery. Surgery is expensive since it needs anaesthetics, sterile conditions and highly trained personnel. It would be much cheaper and simpler if there was no need to cut into the body and cells could be removed without needing surgery. Exfoliative cytology is just such a method of obtaining cells for diagnosis without having to cut into the body.

Exfoliative cytology relies on cells being shed naturally from a surface. These cells can be collected without damage to the body so it is simpler and safer. The commonest form of exfoliative cytology is the use of smears from the uterine cervix to recognize the early stages of cancer (malignancy) but it is also useful for diagnosis of other diseases and for monitoring treatment. Although cervical smears are the most common form of smears they are not the only type and specimens can be obtained from a wide variety of sources.

Use of exfoliative cytology

Advantages of exfoliative cytology

Exfoliative cytology provides a useful alternative to histological examination since it has several advantages when compared to conventional biopsy techniques:

- The collection of specimens is relatively simple and causes very little damage since there is no cutting or incisions. It is considered a non-invasive technique.

- Both specimen collection and processing are quick. Cytology can be used for rapid diagnosis as an alternative to frozen sections. It is easily possible to have a smear ready for diagnosis in a similar time-scale to that needed to prepare a frozen section. Speed is not usually the reason for using exfoliative cytology and most smears are processed as non-urgent and routine reports may take several days, but smears can be processed and reported on within an hour if necessary.

- The technique of specimen collection is cheaper since it does not require expensive aseptic surgery or even getting the patient into hospital. In many cases it can be done during a visit to the GP and it can be done by a trained nurse or equivalent trained personnel and does not need a surgeon.

- Exfoliative cytology can be used as a screening method. Screening involves checking large numbers of apparently normal people for disease in the hope of finding the very early stages of disease in a few of them. It is always easier to treat a disease in the early stages so early detection is of great benefit to the patient and can be cost-effective by reducing the need for expensive treatment of advanced disease. Screening is only possible because of the previous advantages. It would not be possible to screen patients without symptoms if specimen collection was expensive, involved significant risk to the patient or was very painful.

Disadvantages of exfoliative cytology

Exfoliative cytology does have some disadvantages, however, when compared to a full histological biopsy:

- A negative result from a smear is less certain than with a histological section since the cells may reflect a poor sampling of the diseased area and not a genuine lack of disease. For this reason a negative result on a smear should not be allowed to override a clinician's suspicions that there is a genuine disease present. If there is doubt then the smear should be repeated.

Whether to create a screening programme is a complex decision since it involves ethical, economic and social dimensions. The economic decision is the easiest. The cost of screening is compared to the costs of not screening. The costs of not screening includes the extra cost of treating later stages of the disease and the loss of earnings from the disease. The social problems relate to the effects of worry and stress from any false-positives or recalls. The ethical problems relate to how much pressure is used to get people to comply with the screening and whether it is morally justifiable NOT to screen for economic reasons. The aim of the Government is to have at least 80% of women between the ages of 25 and 60 screened for cervical disease at least once every 5 years.

- Even in a situation where a tumour is detected using a smear the actual site of the tumour may be uncertain. For example, if a fluid sample is taken then abnormal cells could have come from anywhere that has come in contact with the fluid.

- The screening of smears can be very tedious. Most of the cells in most of the samples will be normal and screeners can find it very difficult to keep up the concentration needed to detect the occasional abnormal cells. This is especially true for screening samples from healthy people where less than one in a hundred smears may show abnormality and even in the positive cases the majority of cells on a smear may be quite normal.

- The exact nature of the tumour is less certain than when a biopsy is taken since only isolated cells can be seen and their relationship with adjacent cells is lost in the smearing process. Important characteristics such as tumours invading into surrounding tissues cannot be seen directly in smears but only inferred from the appearance of the individual cells.

Because of these disadvantages many pathologists prefer to confirm a positive cytological diagnosis with a biopsy before planning and applying any treatment.

Gynaecological smears

The use of smears for the detection of cervical and endometrial malignancy is probably the best known of all the techniques and has been used for many years. When fully applied it can lead to significant reductions in deaths in the target population. The use of cervical smears as a diagnostic method was pioneered by George Papanicolaou in the 1940s. It was Papanicolaou who developed the main staining technique for smears and the technique is often referred to as a 'Papanicolaou test' and is frequently shortened so that the term 'pap smear' is a common designation for the cervical exfoliative cytology test.

Although the actual techniques of preparing the slides may be identical there are two distinct types of specimen.

Asymptomatic patients

These are collected as part of the cervical cytology screening programme to detect disease before it becomes apparent to either the patient or the clinician. The patients are generally well and the screening is done on a large section of the population. Since most smears are normal the initial checking of these smears is not done by pathologists but by trained **cytoscreeners** who are mainly trying to just separate those smears that are perfectly normal from those that are possibly showing some suspicious signs. The cytoscreeners do not make a final diagnosis though they may indicate the type of abnormality that they find. All abnormalities are marked on the

Symptomatic patients will only really be seen if they go to see their GP with a particular problem. Patients will only visit their GP if the problem is one of the following:

- Painful.

- Worrying.

- Embarrassing.

- Disabling.

Cervical cancer falls into none of these categories until the disease is well advanced and it is then difficult to treat. In the early stages of the disease, when treatment is easy, the signs are quite slight and easily missed. This makes cytological screening essential to detect the early and treatable stage of the disease.

slide (e.g. by a dot of ink next to the suspicious looking cell) and the smears are then passed to the pathologist or cytologist for final diagnosis. All abnormalities are reported and checked not simply malignancy and its early stages. Inflammation and infections are still significant findings and should not be ignored.

Symptomatic patients

In this case there is some clinical reason for taking the smear. The patient may report symptoms or the clinician may detect something during a physical examination. In this case the purpose of the smear is to diagnose the condition and is not just screening. The selection of which cases to investigate is done by the clinician taking into account the symptoms and case history of the patient. The smears may also be used to monitor the effectiveness of treatment. These can often involve more invasive techniques and more frequent sampling since they can be justified by the symptoms. Smears from symptomatic patients should always be seen by the pathologist and not just screened and reported as 'no abnormality seen' since in this case a negative result is not expected and would be considered a significant finding.

The main use of exfoliative cytology is for gynaecological screening

Cancer of the cervix has proved to be a good disease to tackle with such screening. One reason for this is that the earliest signs of malignant change can be seen as simple nuclear changes (dyskaryosis) and alterations in the maturation of cells (dysplasia) in the cervical epithelium. These early changes are not malignant and often subside without progressing to malignancy but in some cases they can lead to further change resulting in a carcinoma *in situ*. This may then develop into an invasive carcinoma if not treated. Table 12.1 shows the typical time course of the disease.

These times will vary with individual patients of course and there is evidence that these time-scales are changing even as an average for the population. Some of these changes are now being seen earlier than was previously the case though the reasons for this altered incidence are still disputed. The pattern, however, remains the same with a significant delay in most cases between the time

Table 12.1   *Typical time course of malignant changes in the cervix*

	Arises at age (years)	Persists
Dysplasia	30	10–20 years
Carcinoma *in situ*	40	5–10 years
Invasive carcinoma	60	1–4 years before symptoms become apparent

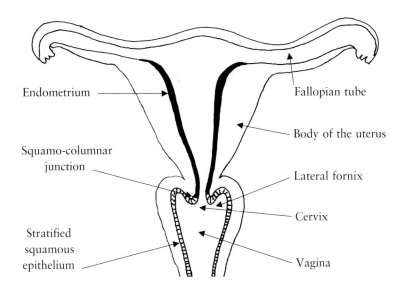

Figure 12.1 *Cross-sectional diagram of the vagina and uterus. The posterior fornix is situated behind the cervix and connects with lateral fornix. The position of the squamo-columnar junction varies so the position in the diagram is an approximation*

when the lesion becomes malignant and the time when it begins to invade other tissues. If each woman is checked every 3–5 years then at least one of the samples should fall in the period between it becoming overtly malignant and the time when it spreads beyond the initial site.

Types of gynaecological sample

The cells for the smears can be collected in a variety of ways (see Figure 12.1):

1. **Aspiration of the posterior fornix.** This technique collects a fluid sample from the vaginal cavity. This was the original technique used by Papanicolaou but has largely been replaced by direct scraping of the cervix or endometrial brushings. The major disadvantage with this method is that the cells have been shed for several hours (up to 48 h) before being collected and fixed. This long delay between shedding and fixing means that degeneration is more pronounced and this makes diagnosis more difficult and less certain than directly sampling the sites.

2. **Cervical scrape.** This is the most common technique and uses a spatula. This is usually an Ayres spatula (Figure 12.2) or one of its derivatives. The original Ayres spatula is possibly not ideal as it does not have a sufficiently elongated tip to ensure penetration of the external os. The cervix should be viewed while taking the smears to ensure correct sampling. This requires the use of a speculum but it is best to avoid using lubricating materials as they can contaminate the smear. The spatula is used to lightly scrape the squamo-columnar junction where the columnar epithelium lining the cervical canal changes to the stratified

Figure 12.2 *Ayre spatula*

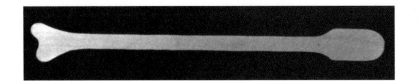

Although cervical cytology is considered non-invasive since it does not break the surface of the body it is not a trivial method of sampling and many women find it embarrassing and undesirable. Getting women to take the test even when it is in their own interests needs good advertising and information systems as well as the scientific ability to screen the samples.

squamous epithelium found in the vagina. The squamo-columnar junction is a very common site of malignant change so sampling of this precise area is essential in screening. The cells are then smeared on to a slide and fixed. Cervical scrapes are the main method of obtaining cervical smears and are usually performed by clinicians, GPs or nursing staff rather than by cytologists.

3. **Endocervical brushings.** The 'brush' can be specially designed or just a cotton wool bud on an applicator. The brush is gently inserted into the endocervical canal and rotated. The cells are then transferred to a slide and fixed. This is less common but will detect endocervical malignancy more reliably and can be used if the squamo-columnar junction is located inside the endocervical canal.

4. **Vaginal wall smears.** These are only rarely done in modern cytology. These were more common in the past when they were used to estimate hormonal status but the use of cytological assessment of hormones such as oestrogen has been replaced by biochemical testing of blood samples which is more sensitive and reliable.

Smear fixation

The smears must be fixed immediately while still wet. Air drying results in artefacts (blurring of nuclear detail for example) especially when the Papanicolaou staining method is to be used, but it is a common method of smear preparation for Romanowsky staining. Many fixatives have been tried over the years but only two are in common use:

- **Alcohol** (95%; sometimes with the addition of 1–3% acetic acid to improve nuclear preservation). This is the usual fixative but the wet solution is flammable and cannot be sent through the post.

- **Spray fixatives.** These consist of alcohols and polyethylene glycols (PEG or carbowax) and the alcohols fix the specimen and then coat it with a thin layer of PEG that protects it from drying. The PEG film is easily removed before staining. These are often bought as ready prepared spray cans or bottles but can be easily made and used from a simple dropper bottle. The advantage of these fixatives is that the polyethylene glycol acts as a protective coating and stops the drying artefact. The slides can be allowed to 'dry' and this is useful for slides that have to be transported or posted.

Staining methods

Staining of smears has to bring out both nuclear and cytoplasmic detail and help to differentiate between the different cell types. Although no single method can be perfect for every situation the Papanicolaou technique has become almost universal in its application for screening of smears. Other stains are more useful for following up abnormalities. Staining needs to be well controlled and reliable since changes in staining are an important feature of diagnosis. Most laboratories would use automatic staining machines to ensure a constant staining routine and to cope with the large numbers of smears being stained.

Papanicolaou stain

The Papanicolaou stain was devised in the 1940s and has been the main cytological staining method ever since. To a certain extent the clarity of this method has been a feature in the acceptance of smears as a diagnostic method. The Papanicolaou method gives good nuclear detail and gives a translucent or transparent cytoplasm that is useful if cells overlap. The ability to see through the cytoplasm of a cell means that it is often possible to diagnose a cell even though there is another cell overlapping it. The cytoplasmic colour gives some indication of the maturation of the cells and of cellular activity. The dyes involved are:

- **Haematoxylin.** Harris's or Gill's are the commonest formulae. Harris's requires differentiation which may result in some unevenness if the smear is thick, but many workers think it gives the sharpest detail when well stained. Gill's is less critical in differentiation and is well suited to automatic staining.

- **OG6.** Orange G in alcohol with tungstophosphoric acid. This stains the superficial cell cytoplasm a distinct but transparent orange colour.

- **EA** (eosin azure). There are several formulations of this stain and they are designated by numbers EA36–EA65. They all contain eosin, light green and tungstophosphoric acid, and the slightly different formulae vary in the light green concentration and whether they contain Bismarck brown and lithium carbonate. The stains do need careful preparation and the commercially available solutions are often used since they give consistent quality.

H&E (haematoxylin and eosin)

This is the most popular stain for histological preparations and is used by some pathologists as it is a familiar technique and matches

It is a little surprising that in three cellular diagnostic disciplines a single stain has become dominant, yet it is a different stain in each case. In histology H&E is dominant, in cytology it is Papanicolaou and in haematology it is the Romanowsky methods. The techniques also do not really transfer across the disciplines. The use of H&E is non-existent in haematology and minimal in exfoliative cytology. Papanicolaou is not used in routine histology or haematology. The Romanowsky stains do have uses in the other two disciplines but only for very limited application. This specialization partly reflects genuinely different requirements in the three disciplines but also reflects a historical inertia. Histologists have always used H&E so they will continue to use it. Papanicolaou has become the most used in cytology partly because it was the first stain in the field.

more easily with histological appearances. Generally the cytoplasmic differentiation is poorer. It is sometimes considered better for specimens prepared by filtering the cells from fluid samples since it is less likely to give a heavy background colour with the filter material.

Romanowsky methods

These are more commonly used for blood smears and as special stains in histology and can be used as a stain for cytology specimens. Giemsa, Jenner, May–Grünwald and Leishman are all examples and which formulation is used is mainly personal preference. The nuclear detail with the Romanowsky dyes is not as good as with a haematoxylin nuclear stain but the differentiation, particularly of non-epithelial cells, is good. Romanowsky smears are usually air-dried and then fixed in methanol rather than the usual wet smear fixation in ethanol.

Shorr's stain

This was the preferred stain for hormone assessment of vaginal smears but is rarely used now as it gives poorer nuclear detail and the cytoplasm is not so transparent as with Papanicolaou. It does, however, distinguish well between the different layers of epithelial cells.

Acridine orange

Acridine orange is a fluorescent stain that differentiates between the DNA and RNA in cells. Since malignant cells tend to stain more strongly for RNA than normal epithelial cells it has been used to detect malignant cells. This method was once proposed as a screening stain for smears and it can be destained and restained (e.g. by Papanicolaou) to allow confirmation by routine microscopy. The requirement for using a fluorescent microscope usually makes it unpopular for routine use.

Stains for special purposes

There are many other stains that can be used for special purposes, e.g. Feulgen (DNA staining) and methyl green–pyronin (DNA and RNA) are used to distinguish nucleoli, plasma cells and Reed–Sternberg cells. Mucins can be stained with the same methods as in histochemistry. Perls technique will demonstrate haemosiderin and asbestos bodies. Gram's stain, ZN and others may be used to detect and identify micro-organisms. PAS or Best's carmine are used to detect glycogen.

Normal gynaecological smear constituents

There are many materials and cells that can be found in normal gynaecological smears. Not all of them will be present in every normal smear, so the absence of certain constituents is usually not significant. The presence of some of these constituents is normal only if they are present in small amounts or small numbers but if they are present in larger amounts then it may be abnormal even though the constituent is considered normal for the purposes of this list.

1. Stratified squamous epithelial cells

These cells all arise from the stratified squamous epithelium of the vaginal or ectocervical epithelium. This is the same type of epithelium that is found in skin. The epithelium is quite robust and resistant to abrasion. The epithelium is multilayered with the cells being produced in the basal layer, maturing in the middle layers and being shed from the superficial layer (Figure 12.3). It is this constant renewal from below that makes the epithelium so resistant. At the base of the epithelium there is a layer of dividing cells.

Following mitosis one of the daughter cells will be separated from the basement membrane and begins to change. The cells become flatter as they mature and they also move gradually upwards through the epithelium as more cells are produced below them. The surface cells are quite flattened and will be lost from the surface with any mild abrasion. It is the upper layers that are sampled in cervical smears and although terms such as 'basal cells' are sometimes used they do not correspond with the very base of the epithelium where the cells are firmly attached and would not be sampled by the relatively mild abrasion with a spatula.

Skin-type epithelium can become keratinized if the upper layers accumulate large amounts of the protein keratin. Although stratified squamous cells in the cervix do have the potential to become

The cervix protrudes into the vagina and on its outer surface and the canal leading from the cervix to the uterus (endocervical canal) is lined with columnar epithelium. The junction between the two varies in life. Before puberty (premenarche) the squamo-columnar junction is inside the endocervical canal. At puberty the cervix enlarges and the squamo-columnar junction is now seen in the vaginal region. This results in a gradual, and sometimes patchy, replacement of the columnar epithelium with stratified squamous epithelium. The stratified squamous epithelium is a more resistant epithelium and is better suited to the vaginal environment. This replacement of the columnar epithelium is called **squamous metaplasia**. The appearance of the squamo-columnar junction in the vaginal region has been referred to by various terms including **ectopy, ectopion, erosion** and **cervical discontinuity**. This is not a disease but a normal phenomenon.

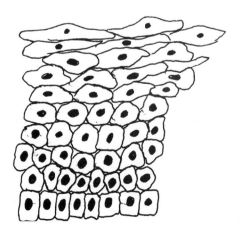

Figure 12.3 *Diagram of the layered epithelium of the cervical surface. The cells are produced in the lowest layer (basal layer) and then gradually move upwards*

keratinized this does not usually happen in humans, though it does in other animals. The distinctions between cells and layers are not rigid since cells gradually change as they mature and the classes of cell are only convenient labels for identifying the stages in cell maturation. Every superficial cell has passed through all the stages and the cells don't suddenly alter but change gradually, so some cells are in between the categories. Some workers include extra types of cell (e.g. precornified) but these are not included in this list.

Superficial cells. These are large (50–60 µm) cells. They have a very small central nucleus that stains very darkly. This condensed nuclear appearance is called **pyknosis** so the nucleus is called a **pyknotic nucleus**. Superficial cells also have an acidophilic translucent cytoplasm (pink or orange with Papanicolaou) which is often angular or 'squared'. This is the most common type of cell in most smears.

Intermediate cells. These are smaller (40–50 µm) cells. They have a larger central nucleus with finely granular chromatin. The cytoplasm is pale green with Papanicolaou and the overall cell shape is angular or 'squared'. Quite a common type of cell in many smears.

Parabasal cells. These are still smaller (20–30 µm) cells. They have a larger central vesicular nucleus with a coarser granular chromatin. The cytoplasm is a denser green with Papanicolaou and the whole cell is rounded or ovoid. This is a less common type of cell in most smears.

Basal cells. Similar to the parabasal cells in most respects. These are even smaller (15–20 µm) cells but have a larger nucleus with a coarser granular chromatin and this may be central or slightly eccentric. The cytoplasm is a dense green with Papanicolaou and is rounded or ovoid. This is an uncommon type of cell in most smears since it is not normally shed from the surface.

2. Uterine columnar cells

Endocervical cells. These cells come from the endocervical canal which is lined with ciliated columnar epithelium. Endocervical cells in smears often vary in how well they are preserved. Cells that are poorly preserved may cause confusion and difficulties in identification, especially for less experienced workers. They are smaller than the squamous cells (15–20 µm). The nucleus of these cells varies quite considerably in size even in normal cells, so variation in nuclear size on its own should not be taken to indicate malignant change. The nucleus is often eccentric usually in the base of the cell. The cytoplasm stains a green-grey colour with Papanicolaou and may contain droplets of mucin in the upper part of the cytoplasm.

The top border of the cells may be ciliated. The cilia themselves can be seen in well-preserved cells but more often only the terminal plate below the ciliated surface is seen. These cells may occur in clumps. In side view the clumps appear as a palisade of cells but in vertical view appear as a honeycomb pattern. Degenerated cells may appear as little more than bare isolated nuclei.

Endometrial cells. These arise in the endometrial lining and are columnar cells but are usually degenerating since they cannot be directly sampled in a simple cervical scrape and may have been shed several days before and then slowly travelled down to the cervix before being collected and smeared. Endometrial cells are small and are only 10–12 μm in diameter. The nucleus is quite large and is usually eccentric with a well-defined nuclear border and often one or two large chromatin clumps may be seen. There is very little cytoplasm and this usually stains a green-grey colour with Papanicolaou but may occasionally be pink.

The cells may overlap or be bunched together. Endometrial cells are only considered as a normal constituent of cervical scrapes around menstruation; significant numbers at other times in the menstrual cycle should be noted and investigated. Endometrial cells may be more common in women fitted with a coil or other intrauterine contraceptives.

3. Blood cells

Erythrocytes. These are easily recognized as they are strongly eosinophilic small cells (7–8 μm) without a nucleus. Erythrocytes are common around menstruation but may indicate bleeding if seen at other times.

Neutrophils or polymorphs. The full name of these cells is polymorphonuclear neutrophil leukocytes but this is usually abbreviated to neutrophils, polymorphs or even just polys. The name indicates their multiple lobed nucleus (*poly* = many; *morph* = shape) which may have from two to four lobes. They are very easy to recognize by their small size and strongly basophilic lobed nuclei. Polymorphs are about 9–15 μm in diameter with a pale green-blue cytoplasm. Small numbers are normal but larger numbers are usually associated with inflammation.

Macrophages (histiocytes). Macrophages are motile cells so they can be very variable in shape and this makes them difficult to identify. Macrophages are larger than other leukocytes (16–20 μm) with a large, lightly stained eccentric nucleus. The colour

> The situation in relation to blood cells is complex since they can represent menstruation which is a normal condition. They can, however, represent disease states such as inflammation and bleeding. Deciding which it is can be difficult and so smears from around the menstrual period should not be used for diagnosis.

of their cytoplasmic staining depends on how active they are and particularly whether they are actively phagocytosing material and the nature of any phagocytosed material. The most common cytoplasmic colour is a light green. The cytoplasm is often vacuolated and may appear foamy if there are large numbers of vacuoles. The vacuoles may contain debris (bacteria, degenerating cells etc.) left from phagocytosed material. Usually only a few macrophages are present in a normal smear and large numbers are associated with inflammation.

Lymphocytes. Lymphocytes are smaller cells (8–12 μm) with a large round basophilic nucleus that occupies most of the cell and there is only a small amount of cytoplasm which is basophilic. They are rare in normal smears and if found in large numbers indicate a chronic inflammation. **Plasma cells** are produced from lymphocytes after they have been stimulated by antigen. Plasma cells have a larger amount of basophilic cytoplasm and an eccentric nucleus with prominent chromatin granules scattered around the nuclear border. This may be referred to as a 'clock-face nucleus'.

4. Other constituents

As well as the cells coming from the epithelia and blood of the woman there are a number of other materials and contaminants that can occur.

Mucus. Mucus is secreted to keep the epithelium moist and prevent the cells becoming desiccated. Mucins appear as translucent strands when stained with the Papanicolaou technique but may stain more strongly with other stains. Only small amounts are usually found in smears and because small deposits and thin films are translucent the presence of mucin does not interfere with cell recognition. If larger amounts of densely staining mucus occur then it will stain more darkly and may obscure some cells and make diagnosis difficult. Large amounts of mucus may occur if there is inflammation present.

Fibrin. Fibrin is an insoluble fibrous protein and is produced from the soluble plasma protein fibrinogen by the coagulation cascade. Fibrin appears as pink strands with the Papanicolaou stain and is usually associated with bleeding. It is normal at around menstruation but at other times it usually indicates a haemorrhage but it can also indicate an inflammatory exudate.

Doederlein (Döderlein) bacilli. These are lactobacilli and are a common commensal organism in the female genital tract. They break down the glycogen that occurs in epithelial cells and release lactic acid as a product of their metabolism. If bacteria are

- **Abnormal staining**. The malignant cells often have quite odd colours. The nuclei may be darker than normal (hyperchromatic), paler than normal (hypochromatic) or stain in different colours to normal (polychromatic).

Cytoplasmic changes

Cytoplasmic changes are less important in recognizing malignancy but the sort of changes that occur include variation in the total cell size, variation in shape of the cell, abnormal cytoplasmic vacuolation and abnormal cytoplasmic staining. Malignant cells may also lose the characteristic features that make them identifiable as a particular cell type. This loss of differentiation is a quite important feature. The less differentiated the cells are the more likely it is that the tumour is an aggressive tumour and is spreading.

Different descriptive terms used to describe the changes

The recognition and reporting of malignant changes is complicated by various factors and varies from centre to centre. There is no absolute test of the degree of malignancy and the diagnosis is made on the basis of experience. Quality control is always in place to check the screeners but there is less check on the final diagnosis which is usually the responsibility of a pathologist.

Malignancy does not happen in a single change but as a gradual development. There is a continuous spectrum of changes from mild changes (which may never progress to a full malignancy) to invasive tumours (which are life-threatening). There are no sharp breaks in this spectrum of changes, so deciding into which category a particular smear should be classed can be difficult.

The reporting phrases also differ even though they refer to the same condition and this may be confusing. There are three main categories of description:

1. **CIN**. This stands for Cervical Intraepithelial Neoplasm and the degree of severity is indicated by numbers CIN1 to CIN3 (three being the most severe).

2. **Dysplasia**. This is a histological description and relates to the changes in cell maturation within the epithelium. Severity is usually indicated by words (mild, moderate and severe).

3. **Dyskaryosis** (originally introduced by Papanicolaou). This is a cytological description of the nuclear changes and indicates severity either using the same phrases as dysplasia (mild, moderate and severe) or by relating it to the cytoplasmic appearance of the cells (superficial cell dyskaryosis, intermediate cell dyskaryosis and parabasal cell dyskaryosis).

Which scheme is used is dependent on the individual laboratory and whichever one is in use it should be used consistently.

The missing of abnormal cells is a serious problem. The target rate for detecting abnormalities is between 85% and 95%. In 1996 there was a case (*The Times*, 6 February 1996) where one laboratory fell below the expected standard and this resulted in the rescreening of 70,000 smears at a cost of £140,000. It was expected that 350 previously undiagnosed abnormalities would be detected though none of these was expected to be full malignancy. However the scale of the problem at that laboratory may have been underestimated. There are reports of five invasive carcinomas, 15 hysterectomies and five deaths in women involved in the screening programme. Many of these women are now involved in litigation against the hospital and the hospital is no longer screening smears.

In 1997 (ironically also the same date; *The Times*, 6 February 1997) a woman was awarded £60,000 following a missed diagnosis which resulted in her losing a child when she became pregnant.

In November 1997 it was revealed that 18,000 smears were to be rechecked in Warwickshire following a low detection rate. Although there have been a series of well-publicized cases of inadequate smear screening it is still better to have the screening than to ignore the possibility of disease. The introduction of computerized screening rather than human screening may eventually reduce the error rate.

My own point of view is that CIN is perhaps a misnomer since the early stages may well not be a true neoplasm and may revert to normal. A condition that can undergo such reversion does not to me merit the use of the term neoplasm. Also the cellular changes seen are assumed to correspond to **intraepithelial** neoplasms but the only way to be sure it is **intra**epithelial is to examine a histological section. This criticism also applies to dysplasia which is a histological description rather than a cytological one.

I therefore personally prefer the term dyskaryosis which is a true cytological diagnosis (it refers to nuclear appearance). I prefer the terms mild, moderate and severe as being more easily understood than the use of cell types.

Within the limits already mentioned the terms do correspond reasonably as follows:

CIN1	CIN2	CIN3
Mild dysplasia	Moderate dysplasia	Severe dysplasia
Mild dyskaryosis	Moderate dyskaryosis	Severe dyskaryosis
		(and carcinoma *in situ*)

The changes that occur correspond to changes in nuclear size and structure and particularly an increase in the nucleo-cytoplasmic ratio. Very early changes which are not sufficient to be classed as dyskaryotic but are sufficiently abnormal to deserve notice (e.g. to arrange an earlier rescreen than normal) may be referred to as 'atypia present' or 'borderline CIN changes'.

Mild dyskaryosis is where cells resemble superficial or intermediate cells by having abundant cytoplasm with angular outlines. The nucleus may show slight irregularities but occupies less than half of the cell. **Moderate dyskaryosis** is where the nucleus is more enlarged and may stain irregularly and the nuclear border may be less distinct and irregular. The enlarged nucleus occupies half to two-thirds of the cell. Finally, **severe dyskaryosis** is where only a thin rim of cytoplasm is usually present. The cell is largely occupied by an irregular nucleus. Sometimes the cytoplasm is larger but there is extra cytoplasm present. The appearance can resemble the nucleo-cytoplasmic ratio in mild dyskaryosis but the nucleus in severe dyskaryosis is actually much larger than in mild dyskaryosis.

The severity of the disease is judged purely on morphological grounds. The number of cells is not significant. A single cell is just as significant as hundreds provided the cytological changes are the same. The number of cells seen to be abnormal is as much an indication of the sampling as of the severity of the disease.

The term **carcinoma *in situ*** refers to the stage when the cells are showing all the cytological signs of full malignancy but they have not yet begun to invade or metastasize. This is a histological diagnosis since it is not possible to tell if invasion has occurred from isolated cells.

The final stage of the diagnostic spectrum is **invasive carcinoma** where the cells have begun to spread beyond the epithelium and

need any specific sugars and most media simply use glucose as the energy source.

- Amino acids. These are the basic building blocks of protein and a wide variety of amino acids needs to be supplied.

- Vitamins. Again human cells cannot synthesize many vitamins which are often essential enzyme cofactors. Individual cells do not necessarily require the full range of vitamins that a complete human being would, e.g. vitamin K is not essential in culturing cells as it is needed for the production of blood clotting factors rather than cellular materials.

- Minerals, trace elements and anions. These are sometimes needed both as nutrients to be included in structural or enzymic proteins and as part of the osmotic and buffering system of the culture medium.

Gases

It is usually appreciated that cells need oxygen since it is the driving force of energy production in the cell but it is less obvious that carbon dioxide is also needed. Human cells produce carbon dioxide as part of metabolism and it is thought of as a waste product but of course in the immediate environment of cells the concentration of carbon dioxide is much higher than in the atmosphere because of the build up from metabolism. The cells are adapted to this level of carbon dioxide and use it as part of their buffering system. Carbon dioxide levels therefore need to be maintained in the medium. Sometimes the medium is formulated to include carbon dioxide as bicarbonate ions and the medium can then be used in ordinary air but some media require the atmosphere in contact with the medium to contain 5% carbon dioxide and cells grown in such media require a special atmosphere of gases.

pH

Cells are very sensitive to pH and must be kept very close to neutrality and will only grow at about pH 6.8–7.4. The pH in the medium gradually changes as nutrients are used and waste products such as lactic acid accumulate. The growth medium is always buffered to minimize these changes using phosphate and bicarbonate buffers but the pH still slowly falls. In order to show the changes in pH the growth medium usually includes phenol red as a pH indicator. Phenol red changes from red (at pH 7.4) to orange and then yellow. So tissue culture media are red at the beginning of the culture and then gradually change colour. Once the orange-yellow colour develops the medium is exhausted and must be replaced.

The complexity of a cell growth medium can be seen from the following formula for 1 litre of Medium 199.

Amino acids:
L-Alanine 25 mg
L-Arginine HCl 70 mg
L-Aspartic acid 30 mg
L-Cysteine HCl 0.1 mg
L-Cystine 20 mg
L-Glutamic acid 75 mg
L-Glutamine 100 mg
Glutathione 0.05 mg
Glycine 50 mg
L-Histidine HCl 20 mg
L-Hydroxyproline 10 mg
L-Isoleucine 20 mg
L-Leucine 60 mg
L-Lysine HCl 70 mg
L-Methionine 15 mg
L-Phenylalanine 25 mg
L-Proline 40 mg
L-Serine 25 mg
L-Threonine 30 mg
L-Tryptophan 10 mg
L-Tyrosine 40 mg
L-Valine 25 mg

Vitamins:
Ascorbic acid 0.05 mg
Biotin 0.01 mg
Calciferol 0.1 mg
D-Calcium pantothenate 0.01 mg
Choline chloride 0.5 mg
Folic acid 0.01 mg
Inositol 0.05 mg
Menadione 0.01 mg
Niacin 0.025 mg
Nicotinamide 0.025 mg
p-Aminobenzoic acid 0.05 mg
Pyroxidol HCl 0.025 mg
Pyridoxine HCl 0.025 mg
Riboflavin 0.01 mg
D,L-α-Tocopherol phosphate 0.01 mg
Thiamine HCl 0.01 mg
Vitamin A 0.1 mg

Osmotic pressure

Osmotic pressure (sometimes called tonicity) again alters during the culturing of cells, mainly due to the gradual loss of glucose and other nutrients. The original osmotic pressure is calculated to include these materials so as they are broken down or incorporated into proteins the osmotic pressure gradually falls. Change in osmotic pressure of the medium is rarely a problem in practice since the medium needs to be changed more quickly for pH changes than osmotic pressure changes, so provided the pH is all right then the tonicity will also be acceptable. Osmotic pressure is usually kept in the range of 280–320 mOsm.

Complex molecules

In addition to the direct nutrients needed for growth, human cells also need hormones, growth factors and other complex molecules to grow properly. These play no structural role in the growth but act as stimulants for the cells. Without such stimulation most cells are not mitotic and will not divide or grow. The complex requirements can be added in pure form but it is common to add a natural source of these as serum (e.g. fetal calf serum) or embryo extracts (made from fertile hen's eggs) which are rich sources of these growth stimulating materials.

Even then some cells will not grow adequately and need further stimulation. Adult human lymphocytes will not enter mitosis unless they are first stimulated by one or more special mitogens. The mitogens used include the lectins phytohaemagglutinin and poke weed mitogen which can be added to the culture medium and will stimulate cell division.

Temperature

Cells are very sensitive to slight rises in temperature and are easily killed at even a few degrees above normal body temperature. Lower temperatures than normal are better tolerated by cells but will greatly slow growth. It is quite usual to handle cells at room temperature for replacing medium, subculturing etc. but it is important to grow cells in a well-controlled incubator. Although cells will tolerate temperature down to about 10°C quite well, they are killed at very low temperatures, e.g. freezing is lethal. It is possible to freeze cells and keep them alive but it requires the use of an antifreeze to protect them.

Sterility

The usual cell culture media are not only ideal for growing human cells but are also ideal for growing bacteria, fungi and other micro-

ures including a generally flattened facial profile, a small low-bridged nose and an extra fold of skin over the eye (epicanthal fold). They also have an enlarged protruding tongue and their mouths are not held closed. They have redundant skin folds around the neck and misshapen, low set ears.

They have a shorter than normal stature and their limb bones are short. The middle phalanx of their little finger is abnormal making it incurving. The palm of their hand shows only a single crease instead of the more usual double crease. They also have an extra-wide gap between the first and second toes ('sandal gap'). Their joints are more flexible than normal. The tone of their muscle fibres is less than in normal muscles and they have pelvic abnormalities.

Mental retardation is probably the single most important feature of the syndrome and Down's patients are one of the biggest groups of mentally retarded people in institutional care. Their intelligence may in some cases be within the normal range but most have an IQ of less than 70.

Female Down's patients have a reduced fertility but any children are usually normal and not affected by Down's syndrome. Males are usually infertile.

They suffer from an increased incidence of certain diseases: endocardial defects 40%; cataracts 2%; epilepsy 10%; hypothyroidism 3%; leukaemia 1%. Alzheimer's disease is common in Down's patients who survive beyond 40 years old.

This is a large list of symptoms so the syndrome is quite complex and involves the imbalance of many genes.

Trisomic fetuses other than Down's rarely survive

Other trisomic fetuses that sometimes survive to birth are those with Patau's syndrome, which is a trisomy of chromosome 13 and occurs with a frequency of around 1/5000 births, and Edward's syndrome, a trisomy of chromosome 18 occurring with a frequency of 1/3000 live births. Most other trisomics abort and do not reach birth. The incidence of most trisomies shows a link with the maternal age (see Box). Other predisposing factors to the incidence of trisomy include exposure to radiation, hypothyroidism, viral infections and familial tendency.

Sex chromosome aneuploidy

The sex chromosomes X and Y have unique features that make them more likely to produce viable aneuploidy syndromes than most of the autosomes.

The Y chromosome is a very small and insignificant chromosome that has no function except for determining sex. The Y chromosome converts the embryonic gonad into a testis and does very little else. The testis then produces testosterone that controls the main body structure and produces either a male or a female type of body.

A number of chromosomal abnormalities including Down's syndrome have a strong link with maternal age. The incidence rises with the age at conception. Mothers over the age of 40 have 20–40 times the risk of having a Down's affected child than a 20-year-old mother. This indicates a non-disjunction of the chromosomes in ovum formation possibly due to the long meiotic prophase.

Girls are born with all the ova in the ovary already partially in the first meiotic prophase. The meiotic division only goes to completion when the egg is ovulated and this means that some eggs may remain in the middle of cell division for 40 or more years. It is hardly surprising that occasionally it results in chromosomes sticking together and not separating. Because of the non-disjunction, one of the daughter nuclei will produce embryos that are trisomic and the other will produce monosomic embryos.

The use of Barr bodies to determine chromosomal sex was introduced into athletics to prevent cheating by men masquerading as women. It was first used in Mexico in 1968. This is at first glance a good test for sex since buccal smears are a better and less intrusive test than physical examination of the external genitals of female athletes, which was the previous method for determining the sex of athletes.

What has happened in practice, however, is that the test has not detected any cheating where men (XY) have tried to compete as women (XX). It has, perhaps unfairly, disqualified athletes who have genuine medical conditions such as XX/XY mosaics and androgen insensitivity. Androgen insensitivity is a condition in which the receptors for the male hormone are abnormal, resulting in the inability of cells to respond to testosterone. Although Barr body-negative (they have only one X chromosome) they are if anything at a disadvantage since they have no response to testosterone (an anabolic steroid) whereas 'normal' women have a low level of testosterone which would enhance athletic performance.

The Y chromosome is, however, dominant and if present will turn the fetus into a male regardless of how many X chromosomes are present.

The X chromosome is large and important and contains many genes totally unrelated to gender. However, in adults only one X chromosome is ever active in any cell. Any extra X chromosomes above the single one that is needed for normal cell activity are 'switched off' during early embryonic life at between day 12 and day 16. This inactivation of any supernumerary X chromosomes is called Lyonization. This results in a visible heterochromatic (dark-staining) structure close to the nuclear border in epithelial cells. This structure is called the **Barr body** and provides a convenient way of determining the number of X chromosomes within a cell.

If only one X chromosome is present (e.g. normal male) then no Barr bodies are seen. If two X chromosomes are present (normal female) then one Barr body is seen as the unwanted X is switched off. The number of X chromosomes is the number of Barr bodies plus one. Abnormal numbers of Barr bodies are found when the phenotypic (body) sex is different from the chromosomal sex, e.g. Klinefelter's, Turner's and 47XXX syndromes.

Barr bodies can be visualized by taking a buccal (cheek) smear and staining with a basic dye such as cresyl fast violet. The Barr bodies are then seen as small, dark-staining structures inside the nucleus close to the nuclear border. Not all cells allow the Barr body to be identified but about one-third of cells should show distinct Barr bodies, so examination of about 30–40 cells should give a good indication of their presence.

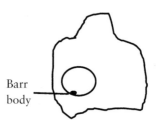

Barr body

Klinefelter's syndrome

This syndrome is associated with an extra X chromosome, giving a complement of 47XXY or less commonly 48XXXY. It can also occur as mosaics in which only some the cells of the body have an abnormal chromosome number. Klinefelter's syndrome has a frequency of around 1/1000 live births so it is slightly less frequent than Down's syndrome. Klinefelter's syndrome patients appear to be male, since they have the dominant Y chromosome, but are usually infertile. Investigation of the infertility may be the first time they are diagnosed and about 10% of all infertile males turn out to be Klinefelter's syndrome cases. Klinefelter's syndrome patients

temperature that is needed (about 0.6°C for every 1% formamide). The balance between temperature and formamide concentration is often the critical factor in controlling the formation of precise hybridization complexes.

Sodium chloride can also alter the stringency of hybridization. High salt concentrations will mask the electrostatic repulsion between probe and tissue DNA allowing less stringent annealing whilst low salt levels will favour very stringent matching. (This masking of repulsion is reminiscent of the salting-on seen with dyes.)

Fragmented non-specific DNA, usually salmon sperm DNA, can be applied to stop non-specific binding of DNA to tissues in the same way that normal serum is used to block non-specific protein binding in immunotechniques. Dextran sulphate can also be used to block non-specific binding.

DNA hybridization is likely to become more important in the future as DNA probes become available commercially. At the present time much of the work being done with *in situ* hybridization uses DNA probes prepared 'in house' since suitable commercial probes are not available. There are some probes available but they do not cover the full range of probes needed. The number of available probes is, however, increasing rapidly. Once reliable probes and simple reliable *in situ* hybridization methods are available it seems very likely that they will be used for many diagnostic situations.

Suggested further reading

Gelehrter, T.D., Collins, F.S. and Ginsberg, D. (1998). *Principles of Medical Genetics*. Baltimore: Williams & Wilkins.

Kiernan, J.A. (1990). *Histological and Histochemical Methods*. Oxford: Pergamon.

Warford, A. (1996). *In situ* hybridization, in *Theory and Practice of Histological Techniques* (eds J.D. Bancroft and A. Stevens). Edinburgh: Churchill Livingstone.

Self-assessment questions

1. Explain what the term cytogenetics means.
2. How can cytogenetics be useful in clinical practice?
3. Outline the preparation of chromosome spreads from human lymphocytes.
   How are the chromosomes made to separate?
4. How can the banding patterns on human chromosomes be demonstrated?
5. Give the karyotype of a normal human female.
   What would a karyotype of 47XY, +21 mean?
6. Approximately how common are chromosome abnormalities at conception and how common are they at birth?
7. Why do alterations in the sex chromosome numbers occur

more frequently than abnormalities in the number of most other chromosomes?

8. What are the differences between the usual Down's syndrome and the translocation form of Down's syndrome?
9. What is a pericentric inversion and how will it affect the individual?
10. Outline the principle of the *in situ* hybridization method. What is its application in histology?

Key Concepts and Facts

Cytogenetics
- Cytogenetics is the study of visible changes in chromosome structure.

- Chromosomal abnormalities are common in human conceptions but most of the abnormal embryos are not viable and abort in early pregnancy.

- Some abnormalities do survive to birth with Down's syndrome being the most common.

- Abnormal chromosomes can be detected by growing the cells in tissue culture and staining the chromosomes during the mitotic phase of the cell cycle.

Abnormal Numbers of Chromosomes
- Euploid variation is an alteration of a complete set of chromosomes, e.g. triploid.

- Aneuploid variation is a change in number but without involving a complete set. Aneuploidy is usually the loss (monosomy) or gaining (trisomy) of a single chromosome.

- Sex chromosomes are more readily involved in aneuploid births than the autosomes because of their special properties.

Structural Abnormalities
- Changes in structure can also be detected, e.g. translocation or inversion of parts of a chromosome.

- Translocations may be transmissible through families, giving familial diseases.

Molecular Genetics
- Molecular genetics involves the identification of specific DNA sequences using labelled DNA probes.

- The probes can be labelled with radioisotopes, enzymes or biotin.

- The hybridization of the probe with the tissue DNA localizes the sites of the sequence.

Chapter 14
Infective agents and amyloid

Learning objectives

After studying this chapter you should confidently be able to:

Outline the limitations of histological identification of bacteria.

List the types of organisms found in sections and name examples of each type of organism.

Outline methods for the detection of micro-organisms in tissue sections.

Describe the nature of amyloid.

List the types of amyloid and their underlying pathologies or physiological conditions.

Describe the major staining methods used to detect amyloid.

Infections of tissue are a common finding in cellular pathology and the ability to recognize the causative agent can be invaluable in diagnosis. Identification from tissue sections is not the best method available and whenever possible identification should be done by microbiological techniques that allow greater sensitivity and accuracy. Most microbiological identification relies on growing the organism and detecting its growth requirements, sensitivity to inhibitors and biochemical tests. Identification from histological sections suffers in comparison to these culturing methods since the organisms are killed by the fixation. Formaldehyde fixation in particular is a very effective method of killing infective organisms. All of the useful microbiological growth methods are lost once the tissue is fixed. Identification of the organism may still be possible but is less certain or more difficult or both.

In infected tissues the causative organism may be relatively uncommon and unevenly spread. This will mean that in an individual section there may be only a few organisms. Unless the staining technique makes these stand out strongly it is easy to miss them altogether. The use of fluorescent techniques (Chapter 15) where the organism is the only material staining against a dark background can help to identify their position in these cases.

Figure 14.1 *Langhan's giant cells. These are large cells, often greater than 200 μm and with a large number of peripheral nuclei. They are found in cases of tuberculosis*

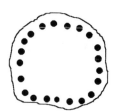

> Accurate identification is often crucial since bacteria are common in many sites. Non-disease causing organisms are called **commensals** and these are common and may even be beneficial. The innocuous commensals need to be eliminated as only the pathogenic organisms are of concern in disease. The rapid fixation of the tissues is needed since many organisms will continue to grow after death and in a few hours or days they can completely destroy the tissue making diagnosis impossible.
>
> The commensal organisms can also mask pathogens by their sheer numbers. One slightly different pathogenic organism in a group of commensals may be easily missed. This can be a problem in post-mortem material where the growth of a harmless commensal may overwhelm the pathogenic organism.

Organisms can also be altered by the processing and care may be needed. The simple staining techniques of microbiologists often need adapting to cope with formalin fixed sections, e.g. Gram-positive bacteria may lose their positive reaction in sections and appear Gram-negative.

Finally there may be the possibility of harmless bacteria proliferating in the tissues unconnected with the disease (see box).

Identification of causative organisms

Although simple histological staining may be limited there is often other information available or other tests that can be tried if a diagnosis is needed. The attempt to diagnose an agent in fixed tissue can involve the following strategies:

- **Clinical diagnosis and symptoms** may be helpful. Often a clinical diagnosis may have already been made and all that is needed to identify the organism is to confirm the clinical assessment. The patient's history may also be helpful in regard of recent travel abroad, ethnic origin, medication and immune status.

- **Appearance of the section.** The body may respond in a characteristic way to certain organisms. Langhan's giant cells (Figure 14.1) are very strongly linked to tuberculosis even if the organism itself is not easily seen in the standard H&E. The appearance of the tissues may not be specific but may limit the possibilities and thus simplify identification.

- **Special stains or histochemical tests.** The stains may be fairly general such as the Gram stain that simply identifies whether it belongs to one particular group or they may be more specific indicating a very limited range of organisms.

- **Immunofluorescent or immunochemical detection.** This method will identify any organism very selectively and can be absolutely specific. The only difficulty is that you can only really use this as a confirmatory method since you need to know which antisera to try. Once you have a very limited range of possible organisms this is probably the best way to identify and confirm an individual organism. The use of immunotechniques is also a good way to spot organisms that are too small to be visualized with the light microscope (e.g. viruses).

- **Nucleic acid hybridization techniques.** These in many ways resemble the antibody techniques in their applicability. Superb as confirmatory methods providing you know what you are looking for. They do have the edge over the immunotechniques in that they will also detect the nucleic acid incorporated into the cell even when no virus particles are present. Some viruses can insert their own nucleic acid into the genome of the host cell and form a latent infection. The herpes virus does this and can regularly break out again causing repeated bouts of cold sores. These latent infections can be quite important and the use of DNA hybridization allows the detection of the virus even when the infection is latent and not active.

Types of micro-organism

Infective agents can be of a variety of types and these vary in their size and life history. Only the major types of organism are dealt with in this chapter though others exist and can be important. Mycoplasma for example are considered to be sufficiently different from the classical bacteria to have their own classification and are important in causing up to 10% of community acquired atypical pneumonia (*Mycoplasma pneumoniae*).

The main groups of organisms are:

- **Viruses.** These are very small and are intracellular parasites. Individual virus particles can usually only be seen with the electron microscope.
- **Bacteria.** These are larger organisms with most being between 1 and 10 μm. Bacteria are visible with the light microscope and a few types can be selectively stained, though not usually positively identified, using simple staining methods. They are probably the most important group in histological identification though not necessarily the most important in terms of disease.
- **Fungi.** These are found in two forms: **yeasts** which are single celled forms and **hyphae** which are groups of cells forming threads. They are often larger than the bacteria and vary from about 2 to 200 μm. They have a distinctively different cell wall to the bacteria.
- **Protozoa.** Tropical diseases such as malaria and sleeping sickness are caused by protozoa. Although once uncommon in Britain, these diseases are becoming increasingly important with immigration and international travel. Some previously minor diseases have also become important in immunosuppressed patients.
- **Helminthic infections.** These are caused by parasitic worms and are more common in countries where hygiene is poor. They are usually quite large and can be recognized by their morphology alone.

Viral diseases are often more difficult to treat than many other forms of infection and so identification may only be of academic interest rather than clinically useful. Viruses can be prevented from causing disease by immunization. This was extremely effective in the case of smallpox which has been completely eradicated by a World Health Organization programme starting in 1967 and ending in 1969 after 2 years with no reported cases. The disease was once prevalent in many countries with fifteen million cases and up to two million deaths. The organism caused a distinctive inclusion body called a Guarnieri body in infected cells.

By contrast there has been a rise in the incidence of human immunodeficiency virus infections but this organism is best seen in cultured cells and cannot be easily identified in tissue sections.

Viral infections

There are many viruses that cause disease and so can occur in tissues. Recognition of viral infections can often be done on H&E sections since they may have distinctive effects on the cells. Although individual viruses are very small they may occur as aggregates where the viruses clump together within the tissues forming **viral inclusion bodies.** The inclusion bodies are rich in both proteins and nucleic acids so they stain very strongly. These inclusion bodies can often be better seen with trichrome stains (Lendrum's phloxine tartrazine) where the differences in acidophilia and basophilia of the inclusion body can be exaggerated. The inclusion bodies often have individual names after the person first describing the inclusion body. The inclusion bodies can be in the cytoplasm (e.g. the Negri bodies in rabies) or in the nucleus (e.g. herpes) or in both (e.g. cytomegalovirus). In some cases such as the surface antigen of the hepatitis B virus (hepatitis B surface antigen, HBsAg, previously also called Australia antigen) there are more selective methods for the inclusion bodies. The HBsAg can be demonstrated by using an orcein stain after permanganate oxidation which converts sulphur-containing protein into sulphonate residues that then react with the orcein.

Electron microscopy is often one of the most useful methods as many viruses have distinctive shapes, though this will often only indicate the type of virus involved rather than the individual species. The use of antisera against the viral proteins is probably currently the best method in widespread use but the use of *in situ* hybridization techniques may become more important as they can be even more specific and have the advantage of detecting viral DNA hidden inside the nuclei of cells.

The **rickettsiae** are intermediate between the viruses and bacteria in that they are more bacteria-like in structure but are obligatory intracellular parasites. Like viruses they therefore produce inclusion bodies in the cell rather than extracellular colonies and so their demonstration in tissues is more related to viruses than bacteria.

Important virus types causing human diseases

Herpes. These are DNA viruses that are often acquired during childhood and then become latent when they integrate their DNA into the host's DNA from where they may re-erupt into active disease in later life. All are similar in structure with a roughly spherical shape of about 120 nm and covered with a lipid membrane. Individual diseases include herpes zoster that initially causes chickenpox but which can re-emerge from latency in dorsal root ganglia as shingles, herpes simplex (HSV1) which gives cold sores, herpes genitalis (HSV2) which causes genital herpes, Epstein–Barr virus which causes glandular fever and cytomegalovirus which often occurs as an opportunistic infection in AIDS.

Retrovirus. These viruses contain RNA rather than DNA and include the HIV virus of AIDS and the human T-cell leukaemia virus (HTLV1).

Paramyxovirus. These are RNA viruses and include the viruses that cause measles and mumps.

Rhinovirus. These RNA viruses include the common cold.

Togavirus. These are RNA-containing viruses and includes the rubella (German measles) virus.

Rhabdovirus. These are RNA-containing viruses and include the rabies virus.

Enterovirus. Although it is best known for its paralysing effects from infecting anterior horn cells of the spinal cord, the polio virus is an enteric virus which first infects the gut and only in some cases does it get into the blood and affect the nerve cells.

Human papilloma virus (HPV). This is a group of viruses causing warts and some types are linked to cervical cancer.

Bacterial infections

The principal method used for bacteria is the Gram stain or one of its modifications. Gram stain detects a difference in the cells of the two types of bacteria though there are several possible explanations. The permeability of the cell wall differs (Gram-positive cells have thicker walls) and this is the simplest reasoning and explains the staining well. The dye (usually methyl violet or crystal violet) penetrates the cell wall and is then aggregated by adding iodine. The large dye aggregates are still easily removed from the more permeable Gram-negative bacteria by a decolorizing agent such as alcohol or acetone but are retained by the more impermeable Gram-positive bacteria. The difference is only in the rate of removal and prolonged washing in acetone will decolorize all the bacteria. The Gram-positive nature does also alter with fixation and processing. Usually a modified Gram stain is used rather than the simple technique but the method is similar.

Some bacteria can be more selectively stained

Mycobacteria can be stained using the Ziehl–Neelsen stain (ZN) for acid fast bacilli. This uses hot carbol fuchsin to stain the mycobacteria followed by differentiation in acid-alcohol. The

Viruses can cause damage to the host in three ways. Firstly the virus may directly damage or kill the cell in which it replicates. This **cytopathic** effect is found with hepatitis A virus that can directly kill liver cells.

Secondly the virus may trigger an immune response in the host. The infection results in viral antigens appearing on the surface of the cell and these initiate an immune response. The result is that the cell is killed and it is the host's response that causes the damage. Since without a host response the virus causes very little damage it allows the development of carriers who have a weak or non-existent immune response to an infection. The host remains healthy but infective, i.e. a carrier of the disease. This can occur with hepatitis B.

Finally the virus may transform the cell into a tumour cell. This can occur if the virus carries an **oncogene** or if it interferes with the cell's gene regulation. The Epstein–Barr virus and some human papilloma viruses may affect cells this way.

The causative agent of spongiform encephalopathy can survive fixation and processing and needs special precautions. The spongiform encephalopathies include Creutzfeldt–Jakob disease and BSE. The causative agent is not, however, believed to be an organism in the conventional sense but an infective protein (prion). The agent can be inactivated by formic acid. There is currently no way of recognizing the agent in tissues and the only identification can be from the characteristic spongy degeneration of the brain.

presence in the wall of these organisms of a hydrophobic material (mycolic acid) is the usual explanation for their retention of the dye. The ability of mycobacteria to resist decolorization is called acid fastness and the organisms can be referred to as AFBs (acid fast bacilli) or AAFBs (alcohol and acid fast bacilli). The acid fastness varies with the species. *Mycobacterium tuberculosis* (which causes TB) is more robust than *Mycobacterium leprae* (which causes leprosy) and will show stronger acid fastness. The ZN technique is often modified to retain the acid fastness by avoiding strong hydrophobic solvents that would extract the mycolic acid.

The technique can also be performed using fluorescent dyes auramine O and rhodamine. This makes it easier to spot isolated bacteria which fluoresce bright yellow against a dark background.

Selective methods have been published for *Helicobacter pylorum* (which can occur in the stomach and is linked to ulceration, gastritis and stomach cancer) and the use of silver staining for spirochetes. Details of these methods are available in many books on technique.

Important organisms seen in tissue sections

Gram-positive organisms

Staphylococcus aureus is a common pathogen and can cause boils, infections in wounds, abscesses and septicaemia. It is a great problem in hospitals where some strains are becoming resistant to several antibiotics (multiple resistance). The clumps of Gram-positive cocci are fairly distinctive. *Streptococcus* species are also Gram-positive but form chains rather than clumps and include *Streptococcus pneumoniae*.

Lactobacillus acidophilus is a commensal found in the vagina ('Doderlein's bacillus'). *Corynebacterium vaginale* may cause cervicitis and is fairly common in cervical tissues (5–7% of women) and *Corynebacterium diptheriae* was once a common cause of disease giving a severe form of laryngitis but effective vaccination has made this a rare disease in modern Britain.

The shape of bacteria and their method of associating together can also be useful indicators of the type of organism present. **Cocci** are rounded whilst **bacilli** are rod-shaped. These two forms are the commonest. Other shapes such as comma-shaped (vibrio) and spiral forms are less common and therefore if seen they can be more informative. If the organisms form chains they can be called streptococci (or streptobacilli) whilst clustering gives staphylococci.

The shape does need to be examined carefully since sections will often slice through the organism so rods can appear as cocci. If there are many organisms present then some will lie entirely within the section and the shape and grouping will be identifiable, but if there are only a few bacteria in a section then it becomes more difficult.

Clostridia species are associated with a variety of diseases including gas gangrene (*Clostridium perfringens*), botulism (*Clostridium botulinum*), tetanus (*Clostridium tetani*) and pseudomembranous colitis (*Clostridium difficile*).

Mycobacteria are also Gram-positive but only weakly so. Although those mycobacteria that cause leprosy and TB are the main pathogenic forms in humans other mycobacterial species may lead to opportunistic infections in AIDS patients.

Gram-negative organisms

The Gram-negative 'gonococcus' *Neisseria gonorrhaeae* is the causative organism in gonorrhoea. The organisms are difficult to find in sections of infected tissues though easier to find in smears. *Legionella pneumophilia* is a small coccobacillus that causes the pneumonia associated with droplets of water from air conditioning units. It has a high mortality rate and is also known as 'legionnaires' disease'. This is again difficult to see in sections. It is easier to stain with silver techniques than with dyes.

The spirochetes are an unusual group of long, slender, spiral, rod-shaped organisms. They cause the diseases syphilis (*Treponema pallidum*) and Weil's disease (*Leptospira interrogans*). The slender rods are difficult to see in sections and need to be stained with a silver technique to see them easily. Suitable silver techniques include Dieterle's, Warthin–Starry and Steiner and Steiner methods.

Fungal infections

Fungi are extremely common organisms in the environment but only a few are pathogenic in humans. The commonest site of infection is on a surface such as skin or in the mouth. The general term for a fungal diseases is *mycoses*. Superficial mycoses such as athlete's foot and ringworm are usually fairly mild diseases but systemic mycoses, where the disease is more widespread inside the body, can be dangerous.

Fungi can occur as yeast or hyphal forms. The hyphae are often distinctive with features such as the presence or absence of cross walls (septae) and degree of branching being useful indicators. Yeast forms are less easy to differentiate on morphological criteria.

Fungi can be stained and demonstrated by the PAS technique which detects their polysaccharide cell walls. Methods using chromic acid as an oxidizing agent (Gridley's technique) or methanamine silver (Grocott's technique) are essentially similar to the PAS technique but are still used instead of a simple PAS.

Important fungi seen in tissue sections

Aspergillus fumigatus is a very common organism in soil and can be a commensal in the upper respiratory tract. If it invades the lung as happens in some AIDS patients it may cause pneumonia.

Candida albicans is found in small numbers as a common commensal in wet mucous membranes but can become pathogenic following antibiotic therapy that kills the normal suppressive bacterial flora. It then causes the condition known as **thrush**. In immunosuppressed patients it can also become systemic.

Cryptococcus neoformans and *Histoplasma capsulatum* can both be acquired from bird droppings and cause systemic disease but are only significant in immunosuppressed patients.

Pneumocystis carinii is again an organism which has only become important in immunosuppressed patients and is a major killer of AIDS patients where it can cause a pneumonia.

The fungal infections were once either comparatively mild and usually superficial diseases (e.g. athlete's foot and thrush) or, if they were life-threatening, they were unusual and often limited to certain occupations. The increase in immunosuppression and immunodeficiency have changed the situation and several once minor or unusual diseases have become common causes of death. In a normal person these infections would be effectively countered by the immune system and either eliminated or kept in check as a low level infection. The loss of immune capability in AIDS demonstrates the importance of the immune system since these diseases have now become killers in AIDS patients.

AIDS patients are said to be **compromised** by the immunosuppression and are much more susceptible to infection and often succumb to minor diseases. The infections are referred to as **opportunistic infections** since they seize the opportunity of growing and spreading in the compromised host.

Parasitic infections

Parasites are large enough and distinctive enough for most diagnoses to be made just on the shape and structure of the organism and the nature of the host's response. H&E staining may be supplemented with a Romanowsky method (such as Giemsa) or stronger haematoxylins (iron or phosphotungstic acid haematoxylin) or a PAS can be used to show glycogen but there are no staining techniques specific for the organisms.

Entamoeba histolytica causes amoebic dysentery and the organism is up to 50 μm in diameter and may contain the remains of ingested blood cells.

Toxoplasma gondii is common in cat litter and can cause an acute inflammatory condition in lymph nodes (lymphadenopathy) but the infection is often unnoticed (subclinical infection). In immunosuppressed patients it can be more dangerous, causing brain infections and inflammation of the meninges.

Plasmodium species cause the various forms of malaria. Malaria is common in tropical countries and is regularly seen in immigrants and travellers. The parasites are usually diagnosed from blood films but they can also be seen in tissues. The associated malarial pigment is similar to formalin pigment and can be removed by alcoholic picric acid. Removal of the pigment allows the malarial parasites to be more easily seen.

Leishmania donovani causes the systemic kala azar whilst *Leishmania tropica* causes the skin disease 'oriental sore'. The infection is spread by the bite of the sandfly and the organisms can be seen in infected areas in the cytoplasm of enlarged macrophages.

Trichomonas vaginalis is found in the urinogenital tract of both sexes. It is commonly seen in smears but less often in sections.

Amyloid

Amyloid is an abnormal protein that accumulates between cells in many organs and can be associated with different pathological conditions. Fresh amyloid has a waxy appearance and absorbs acid dyes though only very weakly. This name is inaccurate as there is no chemical resemblance to starch and it is mainly protein (see Box).

Compostion and structure

Component:	Percentage by weight:
Water and salts	75
Protein (including plasma protien)	25
Polysaccharides (mainly mucins)	1–2
Lipid	0–3

The name amyloid is misleading since it suggests a starch-like material. The eminent pathologist Rudolph Virchow found that amyloid reacted with iodine/ sulphuric acid and produced a blue colour and since this is reminiscent of the blue colour given by starch when treated with iodine he introduced the name **amyloid** (*amylo* = starch).

The later finding that it is protein has led to people suggesting other names but in an attempt to be more descriptive these names have often been clumsy. One suggestion was **idiopathic fibrillar glycoproteinosis**. This name is certainly more accurate than the present one but such names are unlikely to replace the succinct, if inaccurate, amyloid which is much easier to say and remember.

Amyloid protein is a β-pleated sheet

Despite always having a very similar appearance and staining properties amyloid protein is very variable in its amino acid composition. All the different forms have a β-pleated sheet structure and this seems to be the common link between these different materials. Although amyloid has little structure when viewed with the light microscope (i.e. it is **amorphous**) it does form fibrils that are visible with the EM. These fibrils are 7.5–10 nm in diameter but are variable in length and are striated at 10 nm intervals. The β-pleated sheet structure is unusual in human proteins (though it is found in silk) and is very resistant to enzyme degradation, and this probably accounts for its deposition since the enzymes cannot remove the deposits quickly enough.

The different amyloid proteins are related to normal proteins

There are several types of amyloids that have been identified but not all of them are considered pathological. ASc-type amyloid is common in old people but does not seem to be directly linked to any disease. Only two of the pathological types are common (AA and AL) and the others are included for completeness. The two common pathological amyloid types occur mainly as a secondary effect to other diseases and the amyloidosis may be the first clinical finding that indicates an underlying disease. The different types of amyloid have amino acid sequences that are similar or identical to normal body proteins and each amyloid type has a set of diseases or conditions with which it is often associated. Table 14.1 lists the different types of amyloid.

Amyloid P is associated with all amyloids

Besides the main fibrillar amyloid there is a minor protein component that is found in all amyloid deposits, except those in the brain. This component is called amyloid P. It is derived from blood proteins (serum amyloid P, SAP) and is an acute phase reactive protein. The normal blood form of the protein (SAP) appears to bind to amyloid deposits and hence its accumulation, but instead of forming fibrils it forms a 9 nm ring structure made up of five subunits of SAP with a central hole of about 4 nm.

Distribution

Amyloid distribution varies with the disease

Amyloid can occur in many organs and the exact distribution varies with the associated disease. Three types of distribution are often identified:

Table 14.1 *Different types of amyloid*

Amyloid type	Normal protein the amyloid resembles	Diseases the amyloid is associated with
AL Amyloid light chain immune-associated amyloid	Immunoglobulin light chain	Multiple myeloma, Waldenström's disease
AA Reactive amyloid	Serum amyloid A (acute phase reactant, apolipoprotein of HDL)	Rheumatoid arthritis, TB, Hodgkin's disease, familial Mediterranean fever
AE Endocrine related amyloid	Peptide hormones (calcitonin, insulin)	Insulinomas, medullary carcinoma of thyroid
β-Amyloid	Membrane glycoprotein	Alzheimer's disease
AS Senile amyloid		Old age (80 +)
ASc	Transthyretin (prealbumin)	
ASc1	Atrial naturetic peptide	
AF Familial amyloid	Transthyretin (prealbumin)	Familial amyloidosis
AD Dermal amyloid	Keratin	Lichen amyloidosis
AH Haemodialysis-associated amyloid	$\beta2$ micrglobulin	Renal failure with haemodyalysis

1. **Systemic primary**. Amyloid is mainly found in the heart, gastrointestinal tract, tongue, skin and nerves. This is seen in cases of primary amyloidosis and neoplasms of B lymphocytes. The amyloid type is usually AL but this primary distribution pattern can occur with AA amyloid in rheumatoid arthritis.

2. **Systemic secondary**. In this case the amyloid is found in the liver, spleen, kidney, adrenals, gastrointestinal tract and skin. This distribution is associated with cases of chronic inflammatory diseases. The amyloid type that is found is usually the AA variety.

3. **Localized**. Localized tumour-like nodules occur in the tongue, bladder, skin or lung and are associated with localized endocrine neoplasms. The β-amyloid in Alzheimer's disease is also localized but occurs as plaques rather than nodules.

Amyloid can be found in many organs but the frequency with which a particular organ is involved varies and there is no single site that is always affected. Taking a single biopsy sample is therefore never fully reliable as the organ may not be affected in that patient. Common sites include the liver (48%), kidney (87.5%), gingiva (19%) and rectum (75%).

Amyloid accumulates between cells and causes their death

The first accumulation of amyloid occurs between the cells and often close to the basement membranes of a blood vessel. As the deposit increases it gradually infiltrates into tissues and can trap and destroy the cells. There is still doubt about the mechanism of the killing; it may be simple mechanical 'strangling' by cutting off the cells from their blood supply or it may involve a toxic effect of the amyloid. Amyloid has been found to be toxic to nerve cells in cultures but whether it is also toxic *in vivo* is not known.

Effects on organs

Kidney. The amyloid is first deposited in the glomerular mesangium and the basement membrane of blood vessels. As the accumulation continues it eventually obliterates the capillary lumens and destroys the glomerular cells. The amyloid deposit can eventually completely replace the glomerulus. Renal arterioles can also be affected, leading to ischaemia and tubular atrophy. The destruction of the renal tissue produces proteinuria and eventually the **nephrotic syndrome**. Renal involvement is usually fatal.

Spleen. The spleen becomes enlarged (splenomegaly) and the deposits may be of two types: (1) generalized deposits in both the red and white pulp ('lardaceous spleen'); and (2) deposits only in the white pulp ('sago spleen'). If only the spleen is infiltrated and other organs are not affected then it is not usually fatal.

Heart. Usually deposits in the heart are smaller than in other organs. The deposits occur in the subendocardium with more generalized deposits in the myocardium. The deposits may cause pressure atrophy of the heart cells and cardiac amyloid often leads to cardiac arrhythmia.

Liver. The amyloid deposits cause massive enlargement (hepato-megaly) and the liver becomes pale and waxy. The amyloid appears first in the space of Disse and progressively squeezes the adjacent hepatocytes to death. If only the liver is involved then it is rarely the cause of death.

Staining

Since amyloid deposits vary in their composition they will not all stain in the same way. A technique that works well with one sample of amyloid may stain a different case of amyloidosis only very weakly or not at all. A negative staining reaction should be considered inconclusive rather than being definitely negative. If an amyloid deposit fails to stain with one technique then it may be

---

Amyloid deposition has no direct cure but effective treatment of any underlying disease will often slow down or even stop the deposition. Amyloid diagnosis before death has become much more common than in the past due to better biopsy techniques and a greater awareness of the deposition of amyloid. Most patients are now detected in the early stages rather than late in the disease. Whilst this is often beneficial to the patients it has made life more difficult for the laboratories. The large deposits in organs that are easy to find and easy to stain are being replaced with small biopsies containing less amyloid which is difficult to detect.

The deposition of amyloid in the tissues probably reflects a generalized problem with the destruction and removal of large amounts of unusual proteins. The wide range of proteins involved and the relationship with excess protein secretion suggests that during the degradation of the extracellular protein the protein alters its conformation and forms the β-pleated sheet form. The β-pleated sheet form is then more difficult for enzymes to destroy.

If other proteins can similarly change their form during degradation then it is likely that other forms of amyloid will continue to be discovered. There is already a suggestion that in Creutzfeldt–Jakob disease the prion protein may undergo a similar change and produce a specific amyloid type.

worthwhile trying a different one which may give a much better result.

There are a variety of methods that have been used to demonstrate amyloid and some of these are outlined below.

Iodine/sulphuric acid

This method is mainly of historical interest though some pathologists will still use it as a macroscopic method on whole organs while performing a post-mortem. The mechanism is still unclear with the original idea of a carbohydrate in the amyloid acting in a similar way to starch being largely replaced by the concept that it is the β-pleated sheet arrangement that traps the iodine.

Methyl violet metachromasia

Methyl violet has been used for a long time but how it gives metachromasia is not apparent. Amyloid deposits often contain mucinous materials that might explain the metachromasia but methyl violet does not give metachromasia with any carbohydrates or mucins. Amyloid is not metachromatic with other dyes such as toluidine blue that give strong metachromasia with mucins. The results with methyl violet are inconsistent and often difficult to observe. This has led to the suggestion that the methyl violet contains an impurity that is simply more selective for amyloid. This would be analogous to the trichrome methods where differences in staining are relative rather than absolutely selective. It is no longer as popular a method as it once was.

Congo red

This is the preferred method in most laboratories. Most amyloids react and give some staining. The red colour may be weak and some other materials may occasionally stain slightly but it is still probably the best of the current methods. It is even more specific if the section is examined using crossed polarizers in a polarizing microscope (Chapter 15). The amyloid fibrils will show as a dichroic greenish colour. Only chitin and cellulose show a similar reaction and these look quite different to amyloid in sections so there should be no confusion. The section thickness and orientation can be crucial to this colour; too thin and the colour is red, too thick and it becomes yellowish. The fibres need to be oriented correctly relative to the plane of polarization of the light to see the full effect, so only a proportion of the amyloid will be seen at any one time. The rest can be seen by rotating the section. Congo red is also fluorescent so the extent of the amyloid can be seen using this property. (Sirius red is an alternative to congo red for staining amyloid but is not fluorescent.)

Pretreatment of the section with potassium permanganate destroys the congophilia of AA amyloid but AL amyloid is resistant to this treatment so this property can be used to distinguish between the two types.

Thioflavine

This is possibly more sensitive than congo red because of its intense fluorescence but it can be non-specific. It still remains popular as an alternative or complementary method to congo red and is excellent for detecting very small deposits that are easily missed with congo red staining.

Other methods

Other methods include immunotechniques, staining for tryptophan and X-ray crystallography, but these tend to be limited to research into amyloid rather than being reliable and easy identification techniques.

Suggested further reading

Bancroft, J.D. and Cook, H.C. (1994). *Manual of Histological Techniques and their Diagnostic Application*. Edinburgh: Churchill Livingstone.

Francis, R.J. (1996). Amyloid, in *Theory and Practice of Histological Techniques* (eds J.D. Bancroft and A. Stevens). Edinburgh: Churchill Livingstone.

Kiernan, J.A. (1990). *Histological and Histochemical Methods*. Oxford: Pergamon.

Sheehan, D.C. and Hrapchak, B. (1980). *Theory and Practice of Histotechnology*. St Louis: Mosby.

Stevens, A. and Francis, R.J. (1996). Micro-organisms, in *Theory and Practice of Histological Techniques* (eds J.D. Bancroft and A. Stevens). Edinburgh: Churchill Livingstone.

Self-assessment questions

1. Explain why it is better to identify bacterial infections from microbiological specimens than using paraffin wax sections.
2. Outline the types of method that can be used to help identify micro-organisms in tissue sections.
3. What are the major types of infective organism that can occur in sections?
   Name one example in each group.
4. What is amyloid?
   Why is amyloid not destroyed in the body?
5. List the different types of amyloid that are usually recognized and give an example of an associated disease or condition.
6. Name three methods of staining amyloid.
   Explain which you consider to be the best.

Key Concepts and Facts

Infectious Organisms

- Virus particles can only be seen in the EM.

- Viral infections may cause the development of inclusion bodies which can be stained and seen with the light microscope.

- Identification of bacteria in tissues can be difficult as there are usually relatively few organisms in a single section.

- Bacteria can sometimes be stained selectively but positive identification is best achieved with immunotechniques.

- Fungal infections can be stained with the PAS or silver techniques.

- Parasitic infections can usually be seen with a simple H&E or Romanowsky stain.

Amyloid

- Amyloid is a fibrillary protein arranged in a β-pleated sheet form.

- Amyloid accumulates between cells and can destroy tissues.

- Amyloid is often associated with an underlying disease (secondary amyloid).

- The structure of the amyloid varies and is often related to a normal body protein.

- The main similarity between the different proteins is the β-pleated sheet arrangement.

- Amyloid can be stained with Congo red or thioflavine.

Chapter 15
Light microscopy

Learning objectives

After studying this chapter you should confidently be able to:

Describe the principles of simple and compound microscopes.

Describe the importance of numerical aperture and correction of aberrations.

Outline the principles of darkground, polarizing, fluorescence, interference and phase-contrast microscopy.

Outline why the human visual system is not a reliable measuring device and give examples of optical illusions.

Describe how measurements can be made of microscopic objects.

Outline the role of digitization in microscopy.

Most human cells are so small that even a very large cell, 100 μm in diameter, is only just about visible as a tiny speck to the unaided human eye and no internal detail can be seen. Smaller cells, such as erythrocytes or bacteria, are far too tiny to be seen at all. This means that to observe cells in histology and cytology we must use a microscope to make the image larger.

How a microscope works

The size that an image appears to the human eye is controlled by the angle the light makes as it enters the eye. Objects that produce a large angle appear bigger so we can make an object appear larger by altering the angle of light entering the eye. This happens when we get closer to an object and its apparent size increases. Glass, water and transparent plastics can bend light passing through them (Figure 15.1) by **refraction** and this bending can be used to magnify the image. A piece of glass with one or two convex curved surfaces can refract the light to a single focal point and it acts as a magnifying lens or **simple microscope**.

Figure 15.1 *(a) On the left the light ray bends on entering and leaving the glass block. This bending is refraction. In the centre the object is seen as a small structure with only a small angle subtended at the eye while on the right the lens bends the light and makes it appear larger. (b) By bending the light using a lens an object is made to appear larger*

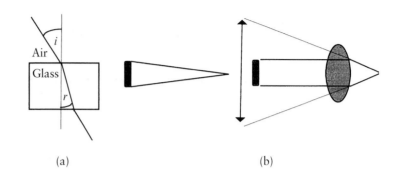

(a)   (b)

The nature of light

Although in most optical diagrams light is drawn as a straight line this is just a convenient way to represent it. Light is an electromagnetic wave and as it travels it is vibrating at right angles to the direction it is travelling. The light has properties associated with this wave nature that are crucial in the theory of optics including microscopy. The important properties for understanding resolution are the wavelength, frequency and amplitude. In Figure 15.2 the amplitude and wavelength are shown.

The amplitude is detected by the human eye as the intensity or brightness of the light whilst the wavelength is detected as the colour of the light. The frequency of the light is the number of vibrations of the beam in one second. Since the speed or velocity of light in a vacuum is constant the frequency and the wavelength of light are linked:

$$\text{Velocity } (V) = \text{frequency } (f) \times \text{wavelength } (\lambda)$$

In the case of light the velocity is approximately 3×10^8 ms^{-1}. Although electromagnetic waves can have any wavelength only certain ones are visible to the human eye. These wavelengths form the visible spectrum of colours and are shown in Figure 15.3.

The wavelength of light varies depending on the medium

When light enters a denser medium than a vacuum it is slowed. Likewise, light travels more slowly in glass than it does in air. The

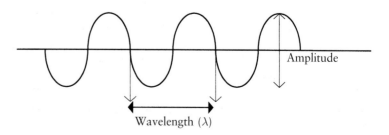

Figure 15.2 *The wavelength (λ) and amplitude of a light wave*

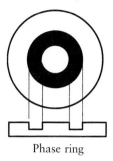

Phase ring

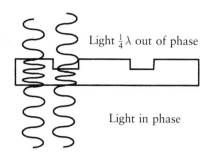

Light $\frac{1}{4}\lambda$ out of phase

Light in phase

Figure 15.18 *A phase ring as used in phase-contrast microscopy. The phase ring is situated in the back focal plane of the objective and consists of a grooved piece of glass. The groove is darker than the rest of the glass. As light passes through the glass the wavelength alters. The light passing through the groove has its phase altered relative to the light passing through the full thickness of glass*

There is much less refracted light than direct light so the grooved area also has some light-absorbing material deposited so that the refracted light and undeviated light have similar intensities and the interference is then more apparent.

Phase-contrast microscopy is relatively cheap as phase plates can be built into objectives fairly simply and will not seriously impair the lens for microscopy when normal illumination is used. It then only requires an annulus to be placed in the substage condenser and phase-contrast illumination is achieved. Substage condensers with rotating filters and annuli are common so that switching from brightfield to phase-contrast or darkground is as simple as rotating a ring on the condenser. Phase-contrast does introduce a distinctive halo that reduces the resolution slightly but the increased contrast it produces in living cells makes it a popular method in tissue culture work.

The differential interference microscope detects phase shifts introduced by the specimen whilst phase-contrast really introduces the phase changes to detect slight changes in refractive index, but in practice they tend to be used in similar ways to look at living cells without the need to fix and stain them.

Photomicrography

The ability to record what you see is just as important in histology as in any other walk of life but to record a microscopic image the usual camera lens is replaced by the microscope and the camera body must be attached to the microscope.

Photomicrography has its own advantages and disadvantages compared to normal photography. The advantages are that for most histological specimens the specimen does not move so exposures can be quite long and this allows slow films to be used. Slow films often have better contrast, better colour rendition and finer grain, so the quality of photographs taken with the microscope can be excellent. The disadvantages are that the microscope is not as versatile as most camera lenses. There is no equivalent of the aperture control which is available on most cameras. This means that there is no control over the depth of field (the amount that is in

The phase ring can be made in the opposite way with a raised platform of glass instead of a groove. This means that undiffracted light is retarded rather than the diffracted light being retarded. This is sometimes referred to as **negative phase-contrast**.

The amount of retardation can also be varied from $\frac{1}{4}\lambda$ through $\frac{1}{2}\lambda$ to $\frac{3}{4}\lambda$. The most common application is for $\frac{1}{4}\lambda$ difference with positive phase-contrast.

The phase-contrast microscope was developed by Fritz Zernicke in 1932 at around the same time as the interference microscope was developed. In more recent years the **modulation-contrast microscope** has been developed. This uses a slit rather than an annulus and a different level of absorption rather than a phase delay. Phase objects are still visualized but the modulation-contrast microscope is better for thick objects and phase-contrast for thin flat objects.

Figure 15.19 *Phase contrast microscopy. Light passing through the annulus forms a ring of light which will pass through the groove of the phase plate. If any light is diffracted or refracted it will pass through the full thickness of the glass and have its phase retarded compared to the undeviated light*

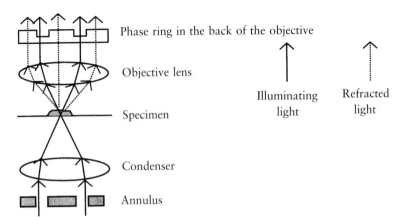

Phase ring in the back of the objective

Objective lens

Illuminating light   Refracted light

Specimen

Condenser

Annulus

Micrography is the recording of microscope images and photomicrography is only one aspect. It is also possible to use drawings to record what is seen. Even in these days of cheap and easy photography the use of drawings still has an important if lesser role.

The recording of very thick specimens in which nerve fibres or similar structures take complex paths through the tissues are still best recorded by drawing. Photographs can only record a single focal plane that can be a very thin slice of the section. The complexity will not be well recorded because of the narrow depth of field. A drawing can integrate several layers of focus into a single drawing and show the full extent of the complexity.

Drawings can also exaggerate differences and become interpretations of the structure as well as a record. The human brain is a very good visual computer and can interpret much better than a camera can record. Drawings are still widely used in books for teaching where interpretation is important.

focus) and exposure is entirely controlled by time. The microscope is also a fixed focus lens so the image cannot be framed differently by moving closer or further away as it can with a normal camera.

There are two types of system used to produce photomicrographs: one is a dedicated system built by the manufacturer to match their microscopes, whilst the alternative is to attach a standard single lens reflex camera to a microscope using a simple adapter.

Dedicated photomicroscopes

The main lens system is in the microscope so the camera is acting as little more than a film carrier and many dedicated photomicroscopes make use of this fact. Manufacturers build systems in which the controls are built into an extension from a third eyepiece in a trinocular head and the film is held in a film carrier that may be a modified camera body or a specially designed unit with no resemblance to a normal camera.

In dedicated photomicrography systems the focusing is arranged so that the eyepieces and the film are in focus at the same time. Since individuals' eyes differ and we can also adjust the focus of our eyes from close distances to infinity there has to be a system to allow for these differences. A focusing eyepiece with a graticule is used to compensate for these variables and the graticule is also used to define the area of the visible field corresponding to the film size. So provided the graticule and the specimen are in focus then the specimen will be accurately focused in the photograph. The light can usually be directed in different directions by moving a lever. The light may be all directed to the normal binocular eyepieces or can be directed to the vertical eyepiece and the camera. Exposure is controlled by opening a shutter for the right length of time. These systems usually have a light meter attached so that accurate exposures can be made automatically. Many have automatic exposure and automatic wind-on so that taking a photograph can be as easy as just pushing a button.

Non-dedicated systems

Single lens reflex (SLR) cameras are a common type of camera that can have interchangeable lenses. With an SLR focusing is done through the main lens and the light is directed into the viewfinder by a mirror. In photomicrography the microscope acts as the lens and all that is needed is an adapter to attach the camera to the microscope. Adapters are usually available from either the microscope manufacturer or the camera manufacturer. When a photograph is taken the mirror inside the camera is swung out of the way and light passes straight through to the back of the camera where a shutter controls the amount of light allowed to fall on to the film. Most modern SLRs have built-in exposure meters to control exposure.

The SLR can be used with any microscope and only needs an adapter so that it will fit the microscope. It is still best to use a trinocular head as it is a more stable arrangement. Focusing is done by looking through the viewfinder of the camera and this also defines what you will get on the film. Focusing can be more difficult using the camera viewfinder and requires the photographer to take his eyes away from the microscope, so there is slightly more effort involved.

The movement of the SLR mirror can jar the microscope causing vibrations that blur the photograph. This jarring was common in early heavy cameras but most modern SLRs are very smooth and do not cause this problem. The use of an SLR is often a cheaper alternative and can give good results. A dedicated system just has a slight edge in terms of quality and ease of use but it can be more expensive. Some high quality SLRs have adaptations that overcome some SLR problems ('swing out' mirrors to eliminate mirror judder, interchangeable viewfinder screens to make focusing easier etc.) but they are also more expensive.

Films for photomicrography

The other important part of photomicrography is the film to record the image. Since most histological specimens do not move there is no need to have very fast exposures. Generally the slower the film the finer the grain of the film, so slow films will capture more detail. Films can be either monochrome or colour. Manufacturers do make specialist photomicrography films but most routine photography is done with the same films that are used for ordinary daylight photography.

Photomicrography is the taking of photographs of small objects and making them bigger. Microphotography is taking photographs of large things and making them smaller. This is done using very fine grain film and has its main use in taking photographs of documents. Many documents need to be stored in detail but are difficult and expensive to keep in their full format. These can be photographed on film and the film takes up much less space. This is done for newspaper archives in libraries where the information is held on microfilm rather than as the full newspaper.

Microphotography is therefore quite different to photomicrography though the two words often get confused.

Monochrome films (black and white films)

Monochrome films are simpler to process and print than colour films but the colours in the specimen are converted to shades of grey in the photograph. This is useful for many journals and newspapers which only print in black and white so it is still quite popular for scientific recording. The loss of colour may mean a loss of contrast since green and red may appear as the same shade of grey. To exaggerate differences the colours can be controlled by using coloured filters. A filter of any colour will make any object of the same colour seem lighter and objects of the complementary colour seem dark. So a red stained cell would appear dark with a green filter (complementary colour) but light with a red filter (the same colour as the cell).

Colour films

Two types of coloured film can be used: **Transparency film** that produces single transparent photographs for projection or **print film** (colour negative) which is used to produce prints. In both cases care needs to be taken to balance the light source to match the film. Most films are **daylight** balanced to match the colours found in normal daylight but specialist films can be bought to match the colours present in tungsten lamps. A daylight film can be used with a tungsten microscope lamp but the lamp must be filtered using a special blue filter to alter the colour balance of the light to match that of daylight. There are too many combinations of light sources, film types and correction filters to be considered in detail. In general it is possible to use correction filters to match light sources and films but careful choice of filters is essential. You need to be aware of the problem and know that you cannot simply put just any colour film into a photomicrography system and expect it to work perfectly without any corrections. It is usually easy to find a friendly expert photographer to give advice and help you get the right balance.

It can also be difficult to get the colour printed correctly by the routine commercial laboratories as histological specimens have very unusual colour mixes. Most laboratories use automatic machines to correct for odd colour casts and they totally misjudge histological preparations. By using a colour slide film it is possible to get an accurate record and then get prints made from the transparencies. This usually gives better colour reproduction.

Optical illusions and microscopy

The microscope is a magnifying system but it is not complete without a something or someone to use its image. In most cases it is used by a human being for visual examination of specimens. The human visual system is therefore part of the optical system.

Number

This is at first sight apparently easy. For example, to count how many cells are dividing all we need to do is take a measured area and count how many cells are in that area. The normal field of view of a microscope is a standard area so it is not unusual to estimate the numbers of objects relative to one standard field. For example, you can count the number of mitotic figures in a high power field to get an estimate of the numbers of dividing cells in a tissue. This is often done but it is only a relative count not an absolute figure. Provided it is only used to see if there are more or less mitoses than usual then simple counting can be useful. If the exact number of mitoses is needed then counting becomes more difficult. The actual number is not only related to the numbers seen in the measured area but also to the size of the objects being measured, the thickness of the section and the distribution of the objects. These are related by the equation

$$N = n \frac{t}{(D + t)}$$

where $N =$ true count, $n =$ observed count ($D =$ diameter of the cells and $t =$ section thickness. However, obtaining an exact calculation requires careful corrections.

Density

Density measurements are again apparently easy but in reality are more difficult. Simply shining a light through a section and reading the result in a colorimeter or spectrophotometer is inaccurate since the distribution of coloured objects is not uniform or even regular. It is the equivalent in a biochemical measurement of not mixing a tube of solution before trying to measure the concentration. The results are not consistent and can be very misleading.

The Beer–Lambert law relates the incident and transmitted light:

$$\log \left(\frac{I}{I_0} \right) = -\epsilon \, dc$$

where $I =$ intensity, $d =$ thickness, $\epsilon =$ absorption coefficient and $c =$ concentration. If the thickness is constant and the material is the same then:

$$\log \left(\frac{I}{I_0} \right) \propto c$$

Since the change in transmission is logarithmic it follows that doubling the concentration does not double the absorption. So if a material has an absorption A such that only one tenth (0.1) of the light gets through when it is evenly distributed. If a section has four separate areas then the following applies.

A	A
A	A

There will be a quarter (0.25) of the incident light falling on each block. Of this light one-tenth will be transmitted (0.025), so the total transmittance is $0.025 + 0.025 + 0.025 + 0.025 = 0.1$:

0.025	0.025
0.025	0.025

and the overall transmission is **0.1**.

If the same quantity of material is concentrated in one sector then the total transmittance will be more (the absorbance will be less) than with an even distribution:

0	0
0	$4 \times A$

The transmittance will be 100% in the three empty sectors but 0.0001 in the sector with all the material:

0.25	0.25
0.25	0.000025

Only the one area absorbs at all and since it is now four times the concentration virtually no light is transmitted through this area but the overall transmittance is **greater than 0.75**, much greater than that in the case where the same amount of material is evenly distributed. Thus in this example the same amount of material ($4 \times A$) can give a transmittance of 0.1 or 0.75.

The only remedy is to measure large numbers of small areas and then integrate the result. This is more difficult and if the areas are small and highly concentrated it may still be inaccurate.

Statistical micrometry

Statistical micrometry does not attempt to directly measure the actual size but attempts to get an estimate of the size and to **calculate how accurate that estimate is**. Absolute accuracy may not be possible but fortunately a high degree of accuracy is not often needed. Since there is wide variation in normal sizes of cells and structures not only between normal individuals but also within the same specimen, then providing an estimate is within a few per cent of the true size it is usually good enough for even the most critical applications in biology. Statistical estimates are not only easier to apply but can give any required degree of accuracy. One example is point counting to measure cross-sectional area.

Point counting

Imagine a carpet with a complex pattern of red and green. If you throw a coin randomly on to the carpet then the chances of it falling on a green part rather than a red part are directly related to the areas of both colours. If the red and green have equal areas then the probability of the coin landing in a green area is the same as for it landing on a red area, i.e. one-half (0.5). If the red area covers three-quarters of the carpet then it is more likely that the coin will fall on the red area than the green. The probability of landing on a red area is 0.75 and on a green area 0.25, the same as their relative areas. If you throw the coin often enough then the areas can be guessed by counting how many times the coin falls on a red area and how many on a green area. This is the principle of point counting.

If a graticule with a large number of dots on is superimposed on a section containing two components, A and B, then the chances of the point falling on A is A/(A + B) (i.e. A/total area). If the number of dots counted is large enough then it is possible to estimate A and B as a ratio and this is the **area fraction** or **area proportion**.

A typical graticule will have 25 or 100 such points. Crosses are often used instead of simple dots as they are easier to locate when seen against a section. Only the centre of the cross is counted and the arms just help to identify the centre point. Using a 100 point eyepiece graticule and a section of kidney the calculation might be something like that shown in Figure 15.28.

Whether the dots fall on an object or not is a random statistical event so it is also possible to get an estimate of the accuracy of the measurement. The accuracy is measured by calculating the relative standard error (RSE). So if an RSE of 1% is achieved then we can be reasonably sure that the true measurement is within 1% of our estimate. The RSE can be calculated from the following formula:

$$RSE = \sqrt{\frac{(1 - \text{area proportion})}{(\text{hits})}}$$

The idea of point counting is similar to that in opinion surveys. Rather than having to ask the whole population what they think about a topic the pollsters ask a thousand people and then extrapolate to get an approximate answer, with about a 3% error. This is quicker, easier and cheaper than asking everybody and is reasonably accurate.

Pollsters do, however, sometimes get it wrong but they do have extra problems in that some people refuse to co-operate and distort the result.

Figure 15.28 *The graticule is used with a section of kidney and in the cortex 16 of the crosses of the graticule are superimposed on top of glomeruli. The area of glomeruli is therefore 16/100 of the area of the graticule. So in this cross-section of kidney the cross-sectional area of the glomeruli is 0.16 or 16%*

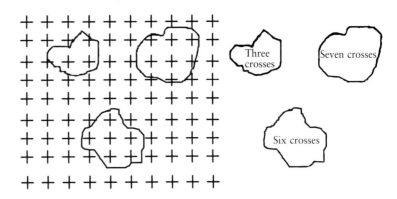

In the case just used the RSE would be:

$$RSE = \sqrt{\frac{(1 - 0.16)}{(16)}} = 0.23$$

This means that the estimate is only 23% accurate. If we wanted 5% accuracy then we would need to count more grids. One single count is not accurate enough. By assuming that the proportion will not change greatly we can tell how many grids are needed. Thus, taking a relative standard error of 5% (i.e. RSE = 5% or 0.05) we use the equation:

$$0.05 = \sqrt{\frac{(1 - 0.16)}{(hits)}}$$

Point counting can be replaced by measuring line lengths across the object but measurement of length is more tedious than simple counting. However, the use of lines can be extended to estimate surface to volume ratio or to estimate complex surface areas or shapes as well as a simple cross sectional area so it is more flexible than point counting.

Solving this suggests that we need to count about 20 grids to get an estimate accurate to 5%. If we need to know the actual areas rather than just the area proportion then we need to know the area the graticule covers on the section and then by proportion we can calculate the actual area in square metres. This area of the graticule can be measured using a stage micrometer.

Volume measurement

Unlike the direct methods, measuring volume with point counting is no more difficult than measuring area. Provided the following conditions are met:

1. the objects are homogeneous (evenly arranged) in the tissues;

2. the sections are thin compared to the objects; and

3. more than one level (i.e. section) is measured – then the following applies:

Area proportion = volume proportion   (theorem of Delesse)

So in the case of the kidney we could estimate that the volume proportion of glomeruli is 16% of the total volume of the cortex. To get the total volume of glomeruli we only need to know the volume of the renal cortex and it can be calculated by simple ratios. In this case we could NOT use the volume of the kidney as a whole since glomeruli are not evenly distributed within the whole kidney; there are no glomeruli in the renal medulla, though they may be reasonably regular within the cortex.

Use of graph pads and computers

Graph pads consist of a flexible membrane covering a grid of fine wires (Figure 15.29). When pressure is applied to the wires they make contact and electrical current can flow through the wires. This is detected by the computer and translated into a position.

By placing a photograph on the pad and drawing around it the outline of shapes can be measured. The accuracy of this technique is limited by the spacing of the fine wires and the accuracy of the operator's drawing ability.

Complex shapes simply consist of a series of X,Y co-ordinates. The length of the lines between each pair of points can be calculated to give the length of a line or perimeter of a closed shape. The graph pad technique still requires calibration but is otherwise extremely easy to use, as the computer can be programmed to do all the hard calculations.

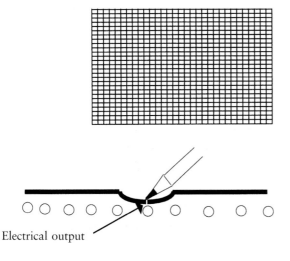

Electrical output

Figure 15.29 *Computer graph pad. A grid of fine wires is arranged with the horizontal wires kept slightly apart from the vertical wires so no current can flow from one wire to the one below it. If the pad is depressed (e.g. by a pencil) there will be electrical contact and current will flow. The computer can then determine which pair of wires are touching and this will give a Y position from the horizontal wire and an X position from the vertical wire*

Figure 15.30 *Diagram illustrating a Feret diameter and convex perimeter*

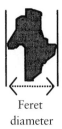
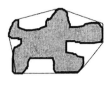

Feret
diameter

Convex
perimeter

Line lengths can be measured by Pythagoras' theorem. For example, inputting two points (X_1, Y_1 and X_2, Y_2):

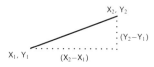

then the distance from the first to the second point is:

Distance

$$= \sqrt{(X_2 - X_1)^2 + (Y_2 - Y_1)^2}$$

With complex shapes there are a variety of parameters that can be measured by simple formulae including:

- area;
- Feret diameters (or 'calliper diameters', see Figure 15.30) where the largest Feret diameter is the length and the smallest is the breadth;
- length/breadth (maximum Feret/minimum Feret);
- convex perimeter (like pulling a string around the shape, see Figure 15.30);
- roundness [$= \text{perimeter}^2/(4\pi \times \text{area})$];
- radius of an equivalent circle;
- convex perimeter [$= 2 \times \tan(\pi 2n) \times \sum n \text{ Feret}$];
- roughness ($= \text{perimeter} \div \text{convex perimeter}$).

Shape parameters such as convex perimeter, roundness and roughness are useful in classifying or measuring abnormalities or shapes which are often difficult to accurately describe in words.

Video digitization is widely used in the film industry to merge computer-generated material with live action shooting, to add or remove objects and to quickly change aspects of a scene without needing to completely reshoot it.

It is also becoming increasingly used in business to automatically read documents (character recognition programs) and for quality control.

The leaders in the field of video digitization are NASA who use video and digitization to send pictures back from space. The Hubble space telescope is a great example of the data collection that can now be achieved with high resolution cameras.

Video digitization

Video cameras have become much cheaper and better in recent years and it is now quite simple to attach a video camera to a microscope in the same way as any other camera. The video images produced can be displayed on one or more monitors or can be recorded on videotape. These systems are excellent aids for microscopy teaching since many people can view the image at the same time. However, they are not only excellent visual aids but the fact that the image is changed into an electrical signal means that they can also be used in measurement.

Television and video images consist of a number of lines that are displayed as a **raster** on the screen by a beam of electrons. The brightness of any line is controlled by a voltage that increases or decreases the number of electrons reaching the screen. By converting these voltages that indicate the brightness of the image into binary numbers it is possible to convert any video image into a string of numbers that computers can use. Each number represents one dot on the screen and is called a pixel ('picture cell') and the image is called a 'bit mapped image'. Bit mapping needs three pieces of data for each pixel:

1. a number representing how far across the screen the pixel is (X position);
2. a number representing how far down the screen the pixel is (Y position);
3. the intensity of the pixel.

Bit mapping is the normal situation for all computer images. A video image from a television source (camera, TV broadcast or VCR) is a single complex electrical signal that varies with time. Such an **analogue** signal needs to be converted into a **digital** form before it can be accepted by a computer. This requires a very fast **analogue to digital converter** and some fast computer memory to hold the resulting data. These converters are commonly called **frame grabbers** or **video digitizers**.

The more pixels a picture has the greater the resolution and detail in the image but the more data that needs to be stored. The intensity data for each pixel may be a single byte or several bytes. Monochrome images typically use only 1 byte (equivalent to 256 shades of grey from black to pure white) whilst colour images typically use more than 1 byte. For colour 3 bytes is common, 1 byte for each of the three primary colours of the display, and this gives 16,777,216 possible colours.

The X and Y positions are not usually stored as separate numbers. Since the pixel values are stored in order as a list the X and Y position of each pixel can be calculated from its position in the list. So the position of the pixel is implied rather than stored in memory.

A 1024×1024 monochrome image will therefore need 1 Mbyte of memory and a colour image will need 3 Mbytes. Many applications do not need colour and monochrome image processing is still common.

Image enhancement

The image can easily be modified to allow the detail in the image to be more easily seen by the human eye. Various techniques can be used to do this, as outlined below.

Intensity shifting

If the image is too dark or too light overall the intensity can be shifted by adding or subtracting a constant from the intensity value for each pixel.

It is difficult to find out exactly how good current technology has become since the most advanced systems are those used by military forces. These are used for automatic recognition of enemy aircraft, tanks and soldiers. The details are classified as secret but it seems likely that they are better than the current commercial recognition systems. When this technology filters out of the secret military area it may well revolutionize microscopy.

Contrast stretching

The difference between grey shades can be exaggerated by using a mathematical operation (e.g. multiplying by a factor or taking the logarithm of the number).

False colouring

Here grey shades are converted into colour differences rather than shades of grey. This uses a **look-up table** to convert each pixel. Each possible shade of grey is simply assigned a particular colour and this is stored as a table of colours in the computer. As each pixel is being displayed the computer 'looks up' in the table the colour corresponding to the value of the pixel (hence the name look-up table) and displays that colour instead of a grey shade. There does not need to be any regularity in a look-up and colours are often chosen to simply look attractive or to enhance contrast. False colouring is quite effective if a particular set of objects can be shown to stand out from the background. If a histochemical test has been done and the colour is fairly difficult for the human eye to see, then computer enhancement will allow the colour to be boosted by using a look-up table.

Inverting

This alters the image from a positive to a negative form.

Measurement and image analysis

The computer can also be used for measurement. A mouse or light-pen can be used in the same way as a graph pad and measurements made in that way. It is also possible to get the computer to analyse the image. This is often complex but commercial programs are available and are becoming more common. Image analysis is now one of the most rapidly expanding areas of computer technology. The analysis is not restricted to histology but is being used in industry, commerce and everyday life.

The application of this type of technology may well revolutionize the whole of cellular pathology with automatic analysis of sections and computer diagnosis. The question is not so much will this happen as when will this happen. The systems are currently too unreliable to diagnose accurately but with the advances currently occurring it would be possible that for some specialist purposes computer technology could be diagnosing sections within a decade or two. They are already used in some laboratories for recognizing chromosomal disorders or screening cytology smears.

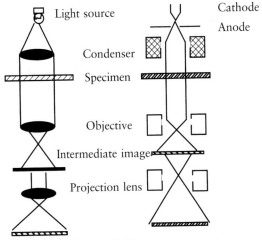

Light source

Cathode

Anode

Condenser

Specimen

Objective

Intermediate image

Projection lens

Final magnified image

Figure 16.1 *Comparison of the light microscope (left) and electron microscope (right). The light microscope is shown inverted for easier comparison. This schematic diagram shows that the two forms of microscopy share many similarities*

condenser focusing the electron beam on to the specimen and extra diffraction and intermediate lenses magnifying and focusing the light after it has passed through the specimen.

Significant differences between the electron and light microscopes

Although there are similarities to the light microscope there are also several significant differences. Some are advantages but some make electron microscopy more difficult and more expensive:

- Electrons have a much shorter wavelength so resolution is improved. This allows high magnification without it becoming empty magnification. Other factors than simple resolving power limit the magnifications used. For biological specimens it is not normally possible to achieve resolutions better than about 10 nm.

- The lenses are magnetic and not glass. Each lens is a coil of wire that generates a strong magnetic field. Electrons are charged particles and so are deflected by passing through a magnetic field; this is similar in some ways to the refraction of light when passing from air to glass. The field can be shaped using **pole pieces** to produce the same magnifying effect on electron beams that a convex glass lens produces with a light beam.

- The shaping of the magnetic field cannot be as complex as the shaping of a glass lens and this limits the ability of lens designers to totally control lens aberrations. To overcome this limitation of magnetic lenses the EM usually works at much narrower apertures than the light microscope since most aberrations are worse when a large aperture is used. Since the wavelength of the beam is so small the reduced apertures do not seriously diminish the resolution and aperture size is less critical than in the light

The apertures in the electron microscope are pieces of molybdenum or platinum with a small hole (200–300 μm) in the centre. This limits the size of the electron beam. The small apertures can be easily contaminated and so become asymmetric. This results in **astigmatism**. This must be compensated for especially at high magnifications. The compensation is carried out with a **stigmator** which is a special multipole magnetic lens that can produce a correcting magnetic field. The control and correction of this is one of the key skills for an electron microscopist. Regular cleaning and polishing of these apertures is an important part of regular maintenance.

The small apertures do increase the depth of field so the EM is actually able to focus more of the thickness in a specimen than an equivalent light microscope lens. The greater depth of field and the very thin specimens used in EM mean that the whole of the specimen can be in focus at once so there is not the constant readjustment of focus needed in light microscopy.

microscope where aperture size (numerical aperture) is the limiting factor in resolution.

- The magnification is altered by altering the electrical current through one or more of the lenses rather than changing lenses, which is the usual way to increase the magnification in light microscopy. Electrons spiral in an electric field, so altering the magnification results in the image rotating as well as getting larger.

- Electrons are easily absorbed or deflected by many substances including air and water. To avoid this absorption the whole microscope tube must be kept in a very high vacuum. The EM requires complex pumps to remove all the air and it must be kept under vacuum since if it is returned to atmospheric pressure the microscope will need to be outgassed for several hours to remove all traces of air.

- Special air locks are needed to put specimens into the microscope without losing the vacuum in the main microscope tube. This slows down specimen changes.

- The specimens must be very thin and dry. This invariably means that EM specimens are dead. There is no EM equivalent to techniques that allows living cells to be examined by light microscopy.

- The intense energy of the electron beam in the high vacuum of the EM can be quite destructive to specimens. Even dead cells need to be well protected by being embedded in plastic to withstand being examined in the EM and unlike light microscopy the plastic is left in place and not removed for staining or viewing.

- Electrons are deflected by any material with a static electrical charge. The specimen is constantly being irradiated with a beam of electrons during viewing and without special precautions this would very rapidly charge the specimen and make viewing impossible. For this reason the specimen must be put on to an electrically conducting copper grid to disperse electric charge and may be coated with carbon to help conduct the charge. The spaces in the grid allow electrons to pass through while the copper bars act as a mechanical support and electrical earth to disperse any static electricity.

- Electrons are not visible to the human eye and must be viewed by using a phosphorescent screen. This phosphorescent screen uses a similar material to the phosphor used in television screens which also use electrons to produce an image. The alternative is to produce a permanent record by using photography. Electrons will directly affect the photographic emulsion so placing a sheet of film in the plane of the image will produce a negative. The EM screen is visible immediately but it is mainly used for identifying which area of the specimen is to be photographed. Photographs are used as the main image in EM as they can be further enlarged

The copper grids used in EM are more intrusive than the glass slides used in light microscopy. It is impossible to arrange the specimens on the grid so it is pure chance where the individual cells lie. The grids all too often interfere with seeing the piece of the tissue that is most interesting. The grids are quite small but have an apparently large area when highly magnified and searching across a grid can seem very tedious. There are no real short cuts since the position is solely controlled by a very fine mechanical X–Y movement. The bars on some grids are made slightly different to allow the operator to know roughly which part of the grid they are observing by giving some 'landmarks' to navigate by.

and are more convenient to view and can be handled (e.g. to measure sizes).

- The image is always a monochrome image. Coloured EM images are artificially coloured often by using computer techniques.

- The contrast between nucleus and cytoplasm and between other structures is enhanced by using heavy metals not dyes. Most dyes will not deflect or absorb electrons sufficiently to act as 'stains'. There are only a few heavy metal salts that are suitable for EM so the range of reagents is more restricted. The fact that only shades of grey are possible also limits the amount of contrast that can be achieved.

Preparation of tissues for the EM

The general principles of histological preparation are similar but the need for very thin sections and the greater detail required in the final preparation mean that there are significant differences in the actual procedures.

Fixation is even more critical for EM

The general principles of fixation that apply to light microscopy are still valid for EM but fixation is even more critical than in light microscopy since subcellular changes can occur within seconds in some conditions. Usually the tissue must be fixed within minutes and becomes almost useless for critical work if left for a few hours. By contrast, post-mortem specimens for light microscopy are often left intact within the body for more than 24 h before the specimen is placed in fixative.

To speed up fixation for the EM the specimen is either perfused *in vivo* or, if this is not possible, it is cut into very small pieces by chopping with a razor-blade. Each fragment may be less than 0.5 mm in size. This allows rapid penetration of fixative. Fixation is often carried out at low temperature to slow down degeneration. Fixatives used in EM include:

- **Osmium tetroxide.** This preserves lipids very well and is the main fixative for membranes and membranous organelles.

- **Glutaraldehyde.** This preserves proteins well and is the main method of preserving cytoskeletal materials.

- **Formaldehyde.** Formaldehyde for EM use needs to be much purer than for simple light microscopy. It is usually prepared by depolymerizing pure paraformaldehyde rather than using the impure formalin solutions that are usual in light microscopy. Since formaldehyde causes fewer crosslinks than glutaraldehyde it is often useful in histochemical techniques and immunological techniques. Stronger crosslinking would chemically alter the tissues, making these techniques useless.

The fixative solution must be carefully controlled for best results

Fixatives can also be mixed to give a compound fixative (e.g. Karnovsky's fixative uses formaldehyde and glutaraldehyde) or the fixatives can be used in sequence to give a secondary fixation (e.g. glutaraldehyde followed by osmium tetroxide). The fixative must be buffered, usually to pH 7.2–7.4 but occasionally higher or lower pH values are used. The buffers used include phosphate buffers, cacodylate buffers and collidine buffers. Some fixatives such as glutaraldehyde may react with some buffers.

The osmolality is also important. Often a slightly hypotonic solvent is used (290–320 mOsm). The fixation time for EM is usually much shorter than for light microscopy, often just 1–4 h, and this is partly a reflection of the much smaller block size which means diffusion is not a major limiting factor. Although fixation is important most laboratories have slightly different techniques which work well in that laboratory rather than there being a single recognized technique used by everyone.

Processing

The waxes used in light microscopy are useless for the CTEM as they would rapidly vaporize in the electron microscope due to the vacuum and electron beam. Instead plastics are used to embed and support the tissues. These plastics can be acrylics or epoxy resins. Acrylics were used in early EM techniques but have largely been replaced by epoxy resins. The use of these materials has already been covered in Chapter 4.

Sectioning

Sectioning of the plastic embedded tissue is done using a glass knife and an **ultramicrotome**. The glass knives are made by breaking a sheet of glass to give a fresh and extremely sharp edge (Figure 16.2). The knives are disposable and have a very short useful life. It may need two or more knives to cut a single block depending on the material being cut.

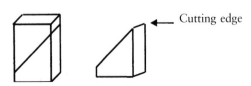

Figure 16.2 *Glass knives. A small rectangle of glass is scored and then fractured to give a triangular knife*

Electron histochemistry

Histochemical techniques can be applied to EM specimens but usually involve **block staining** of fresh tissue followed by embedding and sectioning rather than staining of frozen ultrathin sections on EM grids. 'Blocks' is a very flexible term in EM. A 20 μm frozen section cut in a conventional cryostat can be an EM block since it is large enough to be a complete block for EM. A cryostat section can be cut and stained by a suitable histochemical technique and then processed to produce an EM block.

The final product of the histochemical technique must be electron dense. This occurs with metal salt methods, e.g. Gomori phosphatase methods, and some tetrazolium salts are electron dense (e.g. the osmate of TNST, 2,2′,5,5′-tetra-*p*-nitrophenyl-3,3′-stilbene ditetrazolium chloride). Also, some reaction products (e.g. DMAB product) are **osmiophilic** (i.e. absorb osmium salts) and so will become stained when the block is fixed with osmium tetroxide.

Electron microscopy immunotechniques

These are similar to the immunotechniques discussed in Chapter 10 but using electron-dense labelling instead of fluorescent dyes. Antibodies can be labelled directly with ferritin (an iron-containing protein) or colloidal gold spheres which are visible with the EM. Colloidal gold is probably the most popular since the colloidal gold particles are perfect spheres. Perfectly spherical objects are rare in sections so the positive identification and localization of the spheres is comparatively easy. By using particles of two different sizes to label different antibodies it is even possible to identify the sites of binding of more than one antibody in a single section.

Immunoenzyme techniques are also applicable, e.g. immunoperoxidase, provided the final product can be made electron dense, as is the case with diaminobenzidine used in peroxidase methods which is osmiophilic as mentioned above. The technique can be done either before or after embedding in plastic.

Paraffin embedded material in EM

Although it is usually better to process material directly for EM it is possible to use paraffin processed material as EM blocks. This can be done either from paraffin blocks or from sections.

One advantage is that areas of interest can be identified using light microscopy and only relevant areas are then examined by EM. Since the size of a typical EM section is < 1 mm in diameter this can greatly reduce the number of blocks needing to be examined, thus saving much time and work. Wax blocks simply need dewaxing in xylene, transferring to alcohol and then treating with osmium tetroxide to increase their contrast, and they can then be processed as if they were normal tissues.

The preservation of material for the electron microscope is critical to get the best results but there are occasions when the preservation is poor but it can still be worthwhile looking at the material in the EM. Thus the EM is still a useful tool for archaeologists looking at mummified remains or human materials recovered from bogs. The tissue preservation will be extremely poor but since it is not possible to go back thousands of years to get a better specimen it is better to do the best you can with what you have. Ensuring that fixation and preservation are done properly will always give better results but we cannot ignore the benefits of any technique just because it cannot be done in a perfect way.

Using paraffin sections works best with thicker sections than is usual for light microscopy ($> 7\,\mu m$). The best mode of preparation is to dehydrate the section (to alcohol or acetone) and then invert an embedding capsule containing resin over the area of interest in the section. The resin can permeate the tissue and is then polymerized. The whole thing (glass slide, section and resin capsule) is then cooled in liquid nitrogen and the capsule snapped from the slide. The glass and tissue usually separate very cleanly. The resin block is then trimmed and sectioned.

Preservation of material previously sectioned in wax is adequate rather than good but may be better than tissue stored for several days in routine fixatives. The ability to use sections or blocks is useful in **retrospective studies**. This is where the laboratory has a specimen that could be useful in research in the archives as a paraffin block or section but not as an EM block. So it is possible to do electron microscopy on blocks from many years ago.

Scanning electron microscopy

The scanning EM is quite different to the transmission EM and has no direct counterpart in conventional light microscopy. The SEM is totally reliant on video technology and the user never directly sees the specimen since only a video reconstruction of the specimen is seen on the monitor screen. SEM is mainly used for examining the surface of structures, though by fracturing a block of tissue it is possible to study an exposed surface that was originally an internal structure.

The SEM can examine relatively massive and dense structures since the electron beam does not need to penetrate right through the specimen. Unlike the transmission EM the scanning EM is not often used at very high magnifications; indeed it is quite often used at magnifications lower than when using light microscopy. The main benefits of the SEM are in the way it visualizes objects as three-dimensional photographic images rather than it giving better resolution.

The examination of the surface by the SEM relies on the electrons that are reflected back by the specimen or are emitted from the surface of the specimen when it is irradiated by a beam of electrons. The interaction of electrons with the specimen is illustrated in Figure 16.7.

Electrons produced from the incident beam

The incident electron beam from the microscope produces several types of electrons and also X-rays. The electrons have different energies and properties and will give different appearances to the specimen if they are used to produce the final image.

Back-scattered electrons have a high energy and are produced by electrons in the beam being deflected when they 'hit' an atom in the

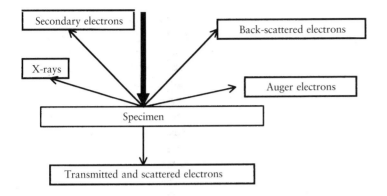

Figure 16.7 *Diagram of scattering of the electron beam*

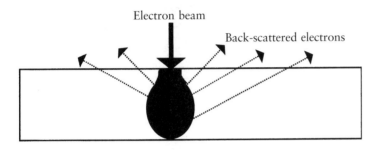

Figure 16.8 *Back-scattered electron production. Electrons are dislodged from a pear-shaped area underneath the electron beam and can escape from quite deep in the specimen as they have considerable energy*

specimen (like a ball bouncing back from a wall). The back-scattered electrons are produced within a pear-shaped region (Figure 16.8) underneath the incident beam and can emerge at quite wide angles. The degree of scattering is partly dependent on the nature of the specimen, i.e. the elements present, so back-scattered electrons give information about the nature of the specimen and not just surface shape.

Secondary electrons have lower energy and are produced by electrons being dislodged by the passage of the main electron beam (like a ball dislodging a brick out of the wall). These low energy electrons can only escape from the specimen from a relatively thin 'skin' (about 2 nm thick) on the surface of the specimen (Figure 16.9). These electrons, therefore, give a good representation of the surface shape. Secondary electrons are less affected by the nature of the material.

Auger electrons are produced by the X-rays interacting with the specimen and have relatively low energy. They are generally not important in SEM.

X-rays and other electromagnetic emissions (cathodelumines-cence and bremsstrahlung) are also emitted but play only a small role in SEM, although they may be used to identify elements present in the specimen.

The main benefit of the SEM is to give quite graphic images of the structures. It is an ideal tool for illustrations in books, images for education and similar visual applications. It is less useful scientifically than the CTEM which shows greater detail and more of the internal structure. The applications of the SEM in diagnosis are quite small compared to the use of the CTEM. There are a few times when it is easier, for example in **hairy cell leukaemia** where the cellular projections are much better seen in surface views than in transverse sections.

There is very little that can be done with the SEM that could not be done, albeit with more difficulty and effort, by the CTEM. Images of the surface and three-dimensional shape can be obtained using replicas and sections taken at different levels.

The SEM image is prettier but the CTEM is more useful.

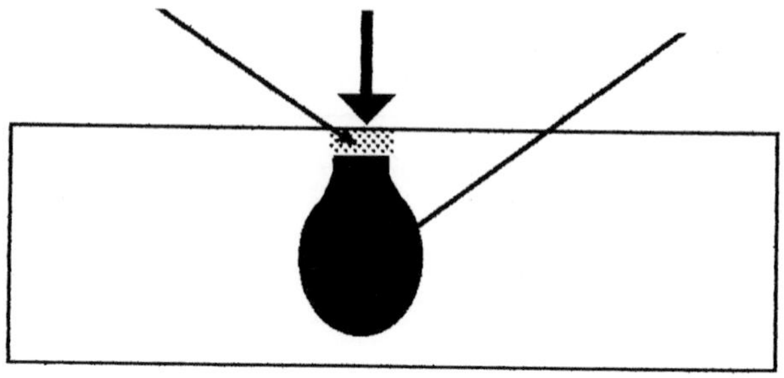

Figure 16.9 *Secondary electron production. Electrons are dislodged from atoms quite deep in the object but their low energy prevents them escaping from the specimen*

Area from which electrons escape

Electron produced here will absorbed and not escape from the specimen

Detection of electrons coming back from the specimen

Detection of the electrons is entirely different to that in the TEM. There is no attempt to focus the electrons to form an image and all the electrons are collected and counted. The image is made by scanning a very narrow illuminating beam of electrons across the specimen. At each point on the specimen, as the incident beam of electrons hits atoms in the specimen, some electrons will be emitted. ALL the electrons are then collected and used to generate an electrical signal. The greater the number of electrons emitted the greater the electrical signal generated. The electrical signal is then used to feed into a video monitor (essentially a high resolution TV system) which is being scanned in parallel with the electron beam in the SEM.

The strength of the signal alters the brightness in the monitor and so an image is built up on the screen, dot by dot as the SEM beam scans across the specimen and the monitor scans across its screen (Figure 16.10).

Higher magnifications are achieved not by increasing the power of the lenses but by the electron beam scanning smaller areas of the specimen. The monitor still displays the same size picture but it now represents a smaller area and this gives more magnification.

Electron collection system

The electrons are collected by a specialized system such as an Everhart–Thornley (ET) collector (Figure 16.11). Other detectors are also available but the ET collector is one of the most frequently used.

The actual detector consists of a **scintillating system** that converts the electrons' energy into flashes of light which are measured by a **photomultiplier** and this produces an electrical signal equivalent to the number of electrons entering the detector. The scintillator is kept at a high potential ($+10$ to $+12\,kV$) so that all the electrons are attracted and accelerated into the scintillant. This accelerating

---

Scintillation is where electrons as they enter certain materials such as perspex emit a pulse of light. The light is weak but can be amplified using a photomultiplier. This instrument converts the light back into an electrical signal. It is ironic that the detectors used in electron microscopy are still employing optical methods and are not purely electronic.

Photomultipliers are one of the most sensitive ways of detecting very weak signals and can detect single photons that are equivalent to single electrons.

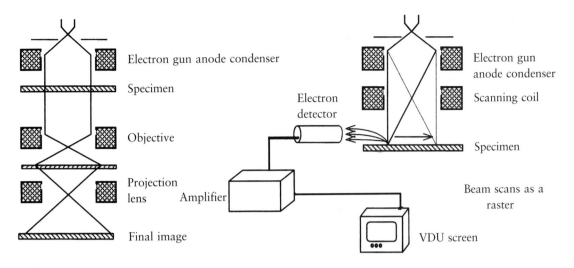

Figure 16.10   *Schematic diagram comparing the CTEM and SEM*

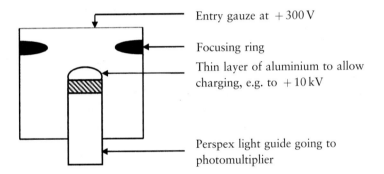

Entry gauze at $+300\,V$

Focusing ring

Thin layer of aluminium to allow charging, e.g. to $+10\,kV$

Perspex light guide going to photomultiplier

Figure 16.11   *SEM electron collector (Everhart–Thornley version)*

voltage means that electrons are collected from a wide area and have sufficient energy to generate a strong flash of light in the scintillant.

An entry gauze is used to shield the system and this is also held at a voltage; by varying this voltage the type of electrons collected can be controlled. If it is held at $+300\,V$ then both back-scattered and secondary electrons will be detected. By altering the voltage from $+300\,V$ to $-100\,V$, or by switching off the 10 kV high tension, the secondary electrons will no longer be attracted but the higher energy back-scattered electrons will still be collected.

The backscattered image is weaker but gives information about the subsurface

The back-scattered image penetrates further into the specimen and is more dependent on the chemical nature of the specimen, but it is also a much weaker signal as there are fewer electrons reflected in

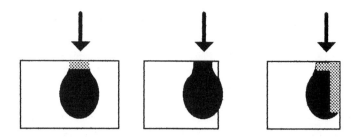

Figure 16.12 *Edge effect in scanning microscopy. The secondary electrons can only escape from the specimen from a shallow region close to the surface but are produced from a larger pear-shaped region below the point where the electron beam hits the specimen. As the beam scans across, the pear-shaped region overlaps the edge of the object (centre). The region from which electrons can escape is now much larger (right diagram) so there are more electrons escaping and this makes the edges appear brighter in the final image*

this way. As a result there is a lot of noise in the image. For most purposes the SEM is only used to detect the secondary or emitted electrons ('emissive mode') which give surface structure rather than penetrating into the specimen. The effect of back-scattered electrons can be reduced by tilting the specimen so that the incident electron beam glances across the specimen rather than hitting it full on and this minimizes the number of back-scattered electrons.

Secondary or emitted electrons give a surface view

The incident electrons penetrate quite large distances (up to 100 μm) into the specimen but the relatively low energy of the secondary electrons makes them unable to escape from deep inside the specimen. These deep electrons are absorbed and lose energy and so are trapped deep in the specimen. The electrons which can escape are those within 2 nm or so of the surface. If there is an edge or hole in the specimen, however, then more secondary electrons can escape (Figure 16.12) and the image is brighter at these points. This gives a 'back-lighting' effect that is aesthetically pleasant.

Some advantages and disadvantages of SEM

Unlike the CTEM the SEM does not focus the electrons coming from the specimen and there are no lenses involved in producing the image, so there are no lens aberrations with the SEM. Despite the relatively high magnifications used in the SEM there is tremendous depth of field (i.e. the image is in focus at both the front and the back at the same time) and this makes for a very pleasing image.

Like the TEM the image is only monochrome but many workers artificially colour the image in order to bring out particular features.

Photographs are taken using a high resolution monitor

Unlike the CTEM it is not possible to use a sheet of film to record the electron image directly and with the SEM photographs are made by photographing the VDU screen. The normal monitor image is relatively coarse so a second, high definition screen is used for making photographs. In this case the scan is performed

The depth of field is impressive when compared to light microscopy. The SEM can take quite large specimens such as complete insects or plants or blocks of wood. The SEM can still show the front and back as being acceptably in focus at the same time even when they are several milimetres apart. The use of a light microscope results in a narrow focus which may be only a few micrometres deep. The only advantage of the light microscope is the use of colour but for monochrome pictures the SEM is better than any of the alternative methods.

very slowly and this gives better definition, but this mode is not useful for direct viewing since only a single dot is visible on the screen and it moves too slowly to allow the human eye to see a complete image. A camera pointed at the screen records all the dots by using a long exposure and so the photograph appears as a complete image.

Since the SEM is used mainly for its three-dimensional aspects it uses whole, intact specimens rather than thin slices or sections of material. Thick sections treated by freeze-etching or freeze-fracture are sometimes used to see internal detail of specimens but otherwise sections are not used in the SEM.

Specimen preparation for the SEM

The usual way to prepare specimens is to completely dry them and then coat them with a thin metal or carbon film to protect them and make them electrically conducting. Electrical conductivity is essential to allow static electrical charges to be earthed. If the specimen is not earthed in this way then, as it absorbs electrons, the specimen becomes highly charged and repels all the electrons before they can reach its surface. Consequently, with an unearthed or uncoated specimen there is no image to be seen.

Specimens are dried and coated for use in SEM

Simple air drying is not recommended since it is uneven and as the water evaporates there are surface tension effects which may damage delicate objects or distort the surface. Instead **critical point drying** is used. Critical point drying relies on phase transitions from a fluid to a vapour without evaporation or boiling. The gas occupies the same space as the liquid so there is no dramatic change in pressure. The phase change can be achieved using CO_2 or Freon, with CO_2 being preferred as it does not harm the ozone layer. The CO_2 changes from a liquid to a gas by a simple rise in temperature. The critical temperature for CO_2 is $31°C$; above this temperature CO_2 cannot be a liquid even at very high pressure and will become a gas.

The specimen can thus be dried without evaporation by putting it into liquid CO_2. Liquid CO_2 is not miscible with water so the specimen is first dehydrated in alcohol or acetone and then transferred into liquid CO_2 in a pressure chamber (commonly called a 'bomb'). The liquid CO_2 is under pressure and is kept below its critical temperature until all the dehydrating agent has been removed. The liquid CO_2 can then be converted to a gas by simply slowly warming it to above $31°C$. There is no evaporation, it just turns into a gas instantaneously without alteration in pressure or volume. The gas can then be slowly released. The pressure is dropped gradually to allow the gas to escape from the specimen in a slow, controlled manner. Rapid drops in pressure will result in

Other forms of electron microscopy and scanning microscopy have also been developed. For example the scanning transmission electron microscope (STEM) which detects transmitted electrons passing through sections rather than the various types of 'reflected' electrons of the SEM, but is otherwise similar in its nature to the SEM.

The atomic force microscope and scanning tunnelling microscope scan the specimen surface using an extremely fine electrical probe. These, at the moment, are much more research tools for particular applications and are often more useful in non-biological fields such as physics and materials science.

explosive escapes of gas from pockets trapped in the specimen which are likely to damage the specimen. The specimen is now dry and can be sputter-coated with a film of metal and is then ready to be viewed in the SEM.

Other SEM techniques

Electron microprobe analysis

The final type of emission from the scanning microscopes that can provide information is the X-rays that are released when electrons are dislodged from their atomic orbits. As electrons move back into the hole created by these dislodged electrons they emit X-rays. The electron shells of atoms are characteristic of each element, so the X-rays produced by the electrons 'dropping' into empty orbits are of different wavelengths with each element having certain characteristic wavelengths. By irradiating one spot with a thin electron beam, as is done in scanning microscopy, and then measuring the wavelength and intensity of the X-rays produced, it is possible to detect any elements present and even to estimate how much of each element is present. This can be done with either the SEM, STEM or the TEM, though the transmission techniques probably give better resolution.

Freeze-etching

In this technique the tissue is first frozen solid and then the surface is dried by sublimation (Chapter 5). This exposes the structure of the dry material in three dimensions. The surface is very delicate and must be protected by gold-coating. The sample is still easily damaged and will not keep. Replicas of the surface can also be prepared for use in the CTEM but the technique is mostly used with SEM.

Suggested further reading

Griffin, R.L. (1990). *Using the Transmission Electron Microscope in the Biological Sciences*. London: Ellis Horwood.

Robinson, G. and Gray, T. (1996). Electron microscopy, in *Theory and Practice of Histological Techniques* (eds J.D. Bancroft and A. Stevens). Edinburgh: Churchill Livingstone.

Slayter, E.M. and Slayter, H.S. (1992). *Light and Electron Microscopy*. Cambridge: Cambridge University Press.

Self-assessment questions

1. How does the CTEM differ from the light microscope?

2. Why do EM sections need to be embedded in resin rather than wax?
3. Why does the SEM not suffer from lens aberrations?
4. What is critical point drying and why is it used in SEM?
5. Why is it necessary to coat SEM specimens with gold?
6. Why is it more difficult in CTEM specimens to identify cellular materials using staining than it is in light microscopy?
7. How can the X-rays produced by the electron beam striking a specimen be used in electron microscopy?

Key Concepts and Facts

Transmission Electron Microscopy

- Electron microscopy gives better resolution than the light microscope since electrons have a shorter wavelength than light.

- Electron microscopes are more expensive to buy and operate than light microscopes.

- Electron microscopy uses magnetic fields instead of glass lenses but is in principle otherwise similar to light microscopy.

- Electron microscopy is more limited in the specimens which it can examine as they must be dry and sectioned very thinly; this makes it impossible to study living cells in the EM.

- Electron microscopy only produces monochrome images and uses heavy metals to increase the contrast.

- Replicas and shadowed specimens can be made by coating the object with a layer of heavy metal.

- Electron microscopy can be used with modified histochemical, immunological and autoradiographic techniques.

Scanning Electron Microscopy

- Scanning electron microscopy uses video technology to produce the image.

- A beam of electrons scans the specimen and reflected electrons are used to recreate an image of the specimen.

- The image shows the surface of the specimen in three-dimensional relief.

- The material does not need to be sectioned but does need to be dried and coated.

Chapter 17

Some aspects of the organization of a histology laboratory

Learning objectives

After studying this chapter you should confidently be able to:

Describe the organization of a routine histology laboratory.

Outline the reasons for storing specimens and data.

Indicate the recommended times for retaining materials.

There are probably as many different ways of organizing a laboratory to produce histological sections as there are actual laboratories. This is in part a reflection of the differing needs and different services. The organization needed to produce a rapid and reliable service for routine diagnosis is not the same as would be needed to produce large numbers of nearly identical sections for teaching. The needs of a research laboratory to be able to tackle problems which may never have been attempted before are quite different to the problems encountered by a contract laboratory which offers a standard level of consistency so that sections will always have the same treatment and a predictable level of quality.

Organization of a routine diagnostic laboratory

There are, however, several features of the organization that are essential and which are common to most if not all laboratories, and the organization of a routine diagnostic laboratory will now be considered in more detail to illustrate the way in which laboratories can be organized.

Specimen types and fixation

Specimens can be of several types and widely different sizes. Specimens that are taken from a living patient are **biopsy** speci-

Answers to self-assessment questions

Chapter 1

1. An artefact is an alteration in tissues brought about by the treatment of the tissue following its removal from the body.
2. (i) Materials normally present in cells can be lost from tissues during processing e.g. glucose. (ii) Materials can be added to the tissues which were not present in life e.g. fixation pigments. (iii) Tissues can be distorted by processing e.g. shrinkage of cells.
3. Glycogen is probably present in the cells since two different preparative techniques show the presence of glycogen. The distribution of glycogen within the cells cannot be determined with any certainty from these sections since the two techniques give conflicting results. One, or both techniques, have introduced an artefact and further techniques are needed to resolve the problem.
4. No single technique is perfect for every specimen and every investigation. Different people have different requirements and each person will choose the method that best matches their needs. Thus frozen sections are good for demonstrating lipids but are not ideal for most routine applications as the tissue cannot be stored easily.

Chapter 2

1. Tissues removed from the body may change by autolysis, where the cells lysosomal enzymes break down the cells structure. Tissues may also change by putrefaction where bacterial or fungal contaminants break down the tissue structure. Tissues may change if the cells remain alive after removal from the body as they will respire anaerobically. Cells will deplete their nutient reserves and the accumulation of waste products may alter the tissues structure.
2. Post-mortem changes can be prevented by stopping enzyme activity. Enzyme activity can be halted by chemicals or heat. Chemical fixation is most common and requires the cells to be treated with a large excess of fixative as quickly as possible.

Perfusion of the fixative through the blood vessels or slicing of the tissue may be needed to ensure rapid penetration to all cells.

3. A good fixative would have the following properties:
   - Penetrate tissues quickly and evenly.
   - Kill cells quickly and evenly, the killing stops abnormal metabolism.
   - Prevent autolysis.
   - Prevent putrefaction.
   - Will not add any extraneous material to the tissue.
   - Does not swell or shrink the tissue.
   - Prepares the tissue for later treatments such as staining and should not prevent any later investigation that might be needed.
   - Prevents desiccation and drying of tissue which would cause shrinkage and distortion.
   - Safe to use (non-toxic, non-flammable).
   - Reasonably priced.
   - Convenient to use (shelf life, storage etc.).

4. Dettol is not a good fixative despite killing bacteria and so stopping putrefaction. The stopping of putrefaction is only one of the three types of change. Only if the chemical also stops autolysis and cellular metabolism without damaging the tissues will it be a useful fixative. Dettol is an antiseptic which can be used on open wounds without killing the tissues and it will not stop normal tissue enzyme activity so it is not a good fixative.

5. Formaldehyde is readily washed out of tissues and leaves no residual aldehyde groups. Glutaraldehyde is a bifunctional aldehyde which is not easily washed out of the tissues so there will be aldehydes from the glutaraldehyde left in the tissues following fixation and these will give a non-specific background reaction with Schiff's method for aldehydes.

6. Fixatives are intended to kill tissues so they are all toxic chemicals. Some are extremely nasty materials and may cause specific problems such as inducing allergies or predisposing to cancer.

Chapter 3

1. Wax embedding is used to support the tissues during the cutting of sections. In the absence of a support medium the sections will collapse and the structure of the cells and tissues will be lost. Wax is the most common embedding medium as it is cheap and allows good sections to be prepared.

2. Fixation (to preserve the tissues), dehydration (to remove the water and replace it with alcohol), clearing (to remove the

alcohol and replace it with a solvent miscible with wax), wax impregnation (to replace the clearing agent with molten wax), blocking out (to set the tissues in a mould with fresh wax) and finally to allow it to solidify to form the wax block. Other steps such as decalcification (needed with mineralized tissues) and vacuum impregnation (not absolutely essential but useful) could also be included in the list.

3. A graded series of any reagent, including alcohol, is where there are a series of baths of gradually increasing strength. The purpose is to remove the water more gently to minimize tissue damage. If tissues are placed directly into 100% alcohol it can cause more hardening and distortion of the tissues than a slower removal using baths of increasing strength. An example of a graded series would be 50%, 70%, 90%, 100% alcohol. Alternatives to alcohol might be acetone, propylene oxide, cellosolve and 2,2-dimethoxy-propane.

4. Clearing agents were so called because they rendered the tissue transparent. This is not true of all reagents but the name has been retained.

5. (i) **Benzene**. Gives good results but is carcinogenic and is no longer used routinely. (ii) **Xylene** is less of a health problem than benzene, it clears tissues rapidly but hardens the tissues and is more useful for clearing sections after cutting than for preparing blocks of tissues. (iii) **Cedar wood** oil is slow and expensive but gives good results. (iv) **Petrol hydrocarbons** are considered safer than many other materials and give acceptable results.

6. Vacuum embedding is the reduction of pressure in the wax bath during wax impregnation and is used to remove air bubbles and help to remove the clearing agent.

7. Mineralized bone can be softened by using acids or chelating agents to remove the calcium salts.

8. Undecalcified sections can be prepared by embedding the tissue in a hard embedding medium such as plastic and then sectioning with a hardened tungsten knife, or by preparing a ground section in which most of the bone is ground away leaving a single thin section.

9. The bone marrow fragments would have lost any mineralized material during fixation as acetic acid is also an effective decalcifying agent. There is no way to be sure if the patient's bones were fully mineralized or if the patient suffered from osteomalacia. (If osteomalacia is suspected then the bone must be protected from acids in the processing).

10. Tungsten knives are harder and can be used for hard and difficult tissues such as bone. They blunt less quickly than steel knives. Disposable knives are thinner and sharper than solid knives but their thinness makes them less rigid and they are not so good for hard materials. Disposable knives are more easily replaced as individual knives are much cheaper so it is easier to

always have a sharp knife. Plano-concave knives have a thin edge profile and are good for cutting soft tissues.

Chapter 4

1. Plastics are harder than most other embedding media and so can be used to cut thinner sections (including sections for EM). They can also be used to cut sections from hard tissues like bone. Preservation of plastic embedded tissue can be better than with wax embedding since plastic embedding involves fewer reagents and does not overheat the tissue.
2. The epoxy resins are preferred for EM since they are stable in the electron beam of an EM unlike wax and methacrylates.
3. Epoxy resins can form bonds with active groups in the tissues (e.g. amines). This prevents dyes binding to the groups and reduces staining. Also the resins cannot be easily removed from the tissues without destroying them so dyes cannot penetrate into the sections and this reduces staining intensity. Neither wax nor methacrylates directly react with tissue groups and can be easily removed allowing dyes to access all stainable groups.
4. The usual way to flatten and remove wrinkles from sections is to float them on warm water. Water soluble waxes cannot be floated on to water as they will dissolve allowing the section to disintegrate.
5. Ester waxes have the advantage that tissue can be impregnated directly from some dehydrating agents. Ester waxes have a low melting point and the lower temperature impregnation causes less damage than paraffin wax embedding. The disadvantages are that ester waxes are more expensive than paraffin wax and they may absorb water during storage.
6. For impregnation celloidin is dissolved in a solvent and the solvent is allowed to slowly evaporate to harden the block. With wax the block is solidified by lowering the temperature.

Chapter 5

1. Slow freezing allows large ice crystals to grow and these can mechanically damage the tissues. Slow freezing also causes concentration of tissue fluids since it is pure water that freezes first. The hypertonic tissue fluids may cause cell shrinkage by osmosis.
2. Frozen sections are used to diagnose malignancy because of the need for an urgent diagnosis. Stained frozen sections can be available within a few minutes of the tissue being removed from the patient. Frozen sections are used for lipid demonstration since the tissues are cut without needing to be embedded or processed. Most lipids are lost if the tissues are processed using organic solvents. Frozen sections are used for enzyme techniques

as frozen sections can be cut without the need to fix or process sections. Fixation will destroy most enzyme activity.

3. In the cryostat sectioning technique everything (tissue, knife and microtome) is kept below freezing so neither the block nor the section thaws during sectioning. In the freezing microtome technique it is only the block that is kept frozen and sections usually thaw during sectioning. The cryostat is better for most purposes but the freezing microtome has some advantages for large blocks or when thick sections are needed.

4. The boiling of liquid nitrogen when coming into contact with warm tissue may slow down the rate of cooling by providing a layer of insulating gas around the block. The use of isopentane, cooled with liquid nitrogen, avoids the boiling problem. The boiling effect does help to prevent minor splashes causing freezing burns to the histologist using the liquid nitrogen.

5. Ice is not completely stable at −20°C and will gradually recrystallize and cause tissue damage.

6. The Peltier module removes heat using the thermoelectric effect. This effect is seen when a direct electrical current is passed across the junction of certain metals and involves heat being absorbed on one face of the module and heat being radiated on the opposite face. The module acts as a simple heat pump.

7. During the warming in a vacuum the frozen tissue loses water by sublimation. The sublimation process absorbs heat (latent heat) and so the block never warms up. The sublimed water vapour effectively carries the latent heat away from the block as quickly as the heat is applied.

Chapter 6

1. Chromophores are groups which bring colour to a dye structure. Without a chromophore group organic compounds are colourless. Auxochrome groups allow dyes to bind to the tissues. Auxochromes are usually ionizable groups which allow the dye to dissociate into charged ions.

2. Basic and acidic dyes bind to ionized groups in the tissues. Basic (cationic) dyes will bind to acid groups in the tissues such as nucleic acids. Acid (anionic) dyes will bind to basic proteins in the cytoplasm and connective tissues. If the two dyes have contrasting colours then they will show the nucleus in one colour and the cytoplasm and connective tissues in the contrasting colour. For example, methylene blue is a basic dye which can stain the nucleus blue whilst eosin is an acid dye which will stain the cytoplasm pink.

3. Altering the pH of a dye solution will alter the ionization of the tissue. If the tissue groups are not ionized then no staining will occur. A high pH will favour staining by basic dyes, a low pH will favour staining by acid dyes. Salts also affect the staining

by altering the ionization and charge on the tissues. At low salt concentrations the ions may help dyes to bind by masking surface charges which would otherwise repel the charged dye molecule. High concentrations of salt are, however, inhibitory to staining as the salt ions will compete with the dye ions for the tissue binding sites. Therefore low concentrations increase dye binding (salting on) whilst high concentrations decrease staining (salting off).

4. With mordanted dyes the mordant acts as a bridge between the tissue and the dye allowing binding. In the absence of the mordant, staining will not occur. If a small amount of mordant is added then it will bind to the dye, forming a dye lake and this dye lake will then bind to the tissues colouring them. If, however, there is more mordant than dye then there will be a lot of mordant without any dye attached. This unattached mordant will compete for the tissue binding sites and inhibit the binding of the dye lake (mordant with attached dye) and so reduce the staining.

5. It is the mordant which binds to the tissue and so it is the mordant which determines where the dye will bind. Aluminium salts bind to the nucleus most strongly whilst other metals will bind to elastic fibres or muscle proteins.

6. The name of the phenomenon is metachromasia. The colour change is believed to be due to polymerization of the dye on the surface of the tissue component.

7. An example of a red nuclear stain is neutral red and an example of a blue nuclear stain is methylene blue. A red nuclear stain is used when the main staining reaction produces a green or blue colour and a blue nuclear stain would be used to contrast with a method producing a red primary reaction.

8. Haematoxylin itself is not a dye and must be oxidized to haematein to stain effectively. The dye solution will improve as atmospheric oxygen converts the haematoxylin to haematein, this is called ripening. The haematein can be further oxidized to a colourless product which cannot act as dye. So a haematoxylin solution will begin to deteriorate when there is more haematein being over oxidized than there is haematoxylin being oxidized to haematein.

9. Dyes differ in their molecular size and their ability to penetrate is dependent on this size. Small molecules will penetrate more readily than larger dyes. When in direct competition the larger dyes will tend to displace or mask the smaller, paler dyes. Tissues differ in their permeability with red cells being very dense, most cytoplasm being intermediate and collagen being very permeable. Using a small yellow or orange dye, an intermediate-sized red dye and a large blue dye it is possible to arrange conditions so that only the smallest dye will stain the dense red cells and they will stain yellow or orange. The medium dye and small dye will both be able to penetrate and

stain the specimen without interfering with the fluorescence of the fluorescein.

4. Alkaline phosphatase and horse radish peroxidase are two enzymes used in immunocytochemistry.

5. For the peroxidase–anti–peroxidase method the following steps are needed:
    (i) Bring test sections to water.
    (ii) Treat with diluted primary antibody.
    (iii) Wash well to remove excess antibody.
    (iv) Treat with bridging antibody.
    (v) Wash well to remove excess bridging antibody.
    (vi) Treat with PAP reagent.
    (vii) Wash well to remove excess PAP.
    (viii) Incubate in enzyme substrate solution to detect sites of binding.
    (ix) Counterstain.
    (x) Sections are finally mounted.
   In addition to these steps it may be necessary to destroy any endogenous peroxidase activity and to prevent non-specific binding by blocking with normal (non-immune) sera. It may also be necessary to unmask antigens. These three extra steps would normally be done before step ii.

6. The final product of the PAP technique is the brown deposit from DAB and this can be treated with osmium tetroxide which makes it visible with the EM.

7. Antigen retrieval is the treatment of sections to allow the antigens to be available to the antibody. This may be needed after some fixation and processing schedules. Antigen retrieval can be done using proteolytic enzymes, microwave heating or heating in a pressure cooker.

8. Lectins can be labelled using fluorescein, enzymes, gold particles etc. in the same way as antibodies. The lectins will bind to specific carbohydrates in tissue and can be visualized in the same way as for antibodies.

9. It is mainly used in EM where the colloidal gold particles are easily recognizable.

10. Avidin is a high affinity binding agent for biotin. Avidin can be used to bridge between biotin labelled antibodies and biotin labelled enzymes.

Chapter 11

1. Autoradiography uses chemicals labelled with radioisotopes. The position of the radioisotopes can be determined by using a photographic emulsion. When the radioisotopes decay the ionizing radiations affect the film. After development the areas of the emulsion exposed to the ionizing radiations show black and this locates the radioisotopes.

2. The prostaglandin will be removed by hydrophobic solvents, but since it will be bound to a receptor and has a low solubility in water it is likely to withstand freezing and thawing without being displaced. Therefore the tissue can be cut as unfixed cryostat sections which can then be air dried. The dry sections can then be coated in emulsion. A dipping technique would be suitable since there is no indication that accurate quantitation is needed but a stripping technique would also be appropriate and it would depend on which was most readily available. Following successful exposure the slide could be stained with a standard H&E.

3. (a) Two possibilities using ^{14}C ($^{14}C_2H_5OH$) or ^3H ($C_2^3H_5OH$). (b) The labelling could be on the sulphur ^{35}S ($H^{35}SCH_2CH(NH_2)CO_2H$), or any of the carbons could be labelled with ^{14}C or using tritium it would be reasonable to label the three hydrogens directly attached to a carbon ($HSC^3H_2C^3H(NH_2)CO_2H$). (c) Labelling here is not very reliable with any atoms. Oxygen has no suitable radioisotopes and labelling the H with tritium is not likely to be stable so autoradiography is possibly not the best technique. (d) Only the phosphorus is suitable ($H_3{}^{32}PO_4$).

4. Dipping techniques are cheaper and quicker for large numbers of specimens. Stripping film techniques are more reproducible for quantitation.

5. Fogging is the blackening of the film at a point not affected by the radioisotopes used in the experiment. This non-specific blackening can be due to chemical contamination, exposure to light, stray radiation from another source (e.g. cosmic rays) or pressure on the film.

Chapter 12

1. Any method used for screening must not have any serious risk for the patient, it must not be painful for the patient and must be reasonably inexpensive. Exfoliative cytology uses only cells being naturally shed from the body and so does not seriously damage the patient. Cervical cytology sampling should not be painful though patients may consider it uncomfortable or embarrassing. It is not too expensive as it can be performed by GPs or nurses without the need for a hospital appointment or full surgery.

2. Endometrial smears are taken from inside the endocervical canal using a swab or brush. Cervical smears sample the squamo–columnar junction at the lower end of the cervix using a specially shaped spatula. Vaginal smears are taken from the wall of the vagina using a simple spatula. Cervical smears are the common form and vaginal smears are now uncommon.

3. The main method of staining gynaecological smears is the Papanicolaou method. This method gives good nuclear detail, transparent cytoplasm and good cytoplasmic differentiation between the different cell layers. Other methods do not have this range of properties though they may be useful in more specific cases.

4. (a) Superficial cells are normal constituents of smears. (b) Parabasal cells are unusual but not abnormal constituents of smears and are more common when oestrogen levels are lowered. (c) *Trichomonas vaginalis* is a pathogenic organism though in some patients it may not cause any symptoms. (d) Dyskaryotic cells are abnormal though mild dyskaryosis may revert to normal. (e) Koilocytes are indicative of viral infection and are not normal. (f) Erythrocytes are normal at around menstruation but at other times they indicate a haemorrhage. (g) Plasma cells are uncommon in normal smears and usually indicate a chronic inflammation.

5. A navicular cell shows an elongation of the cells with curling edges giving a boat shaped cell with an eccentric nucleus. This is usually found in pregnancy.

6. The best stages to take smears are around ovulation i.e. late proliferative phase, ovulatory phase and early secretory phase. Smears taken around menstruation are unsuitable.

7. Acute inflammation will typically show a large increase in the numbers of neutrophils present, with possibly more mucin and sometimes the presence of fibrin and red blood cells from a haemorrhage. If there is an infection then the characteristic organisms may be seen and the cells may show signs of degeneration. Chronic inflammation will typically show an increase in macrophages and lymphocytes rather than the neutrophil leukocytosis.

8. *Trichomonas vaginalis*, *Candida albicans*, herpes virus, human papilloma virus.

9. Cervical intraepithelial neoplasm.

10. Too few cells in the smear, lack of endocervical cells in the smear, presence of red cells which are obscuring detail, presence of pus which is obscuring detail and air drying or inadequate fixation.

Chapter 13

1. Cytogenetics is the study of changes in chromosome number or structure which can be seen by microscopy.

2. Cytogenetics can diagnose syndromes associated with chromosomal changes before and after birth. Although diagnosis in children and adults cannot lead to the disease being cured (the abnormalities are currently not curable) the recognition of a genetic abnormality will allow treatment of the symptoms and

save the need for further diagnostic investigation. Prenatal diagnosis allows the possibility of termination of the pregnancy to avoid the birth of a severely affected child. Cytogenetics can also be of help in diagnosing somatic diseases such as leukaemia where there may be characteristic chromosomal changes in the diseased cells.

3. Cells are taken from the patient (blood cells, chorionic villus cells or amniocentesis cell samples) and grown in culture. Cells may need to be stimulated to divide in some cases and cells may be treated with colchicine to accumulate mitotic cells. Cells are then treated with hypotonic solutions, fixed and spread onto a slide and finally stained to show banding. The hypotonic solution causes the cells to absorb water by osmosis and this inflates the cells and causes the chromosomes to separate.

4. The banding patterns can be stained by using fluorescent dyes such as quinacrine or by Giemsa staining following digestion of the cells.

5. A normal female has the constitution 46XX. 47XY, +21 would indicate a male Down's patient.

6. At conception it is estimated that up to 1 in 12 (~7.5%) human conceptions are chromosomally abnormal and this falls to about 1 in 200 (~at birth. 0.6%) due to spontaneous abortions.

7. The Y chromosome is small and contains only genes needed by a male fetus. The absence of a Y chromosome simply results in the female phenotype being produced. The presence of an extra Y carries few extra genes and seems to cause only minor physiological consequences. The cells have a mechanism to switch off any X chromosomes in excess of the single X found in males, to maintain the chromosome balance between the different sexes. This means that supernumerary X chromosomes do not cause the severe abnormalities seen with comparably sized autosomes.

8. In translocation Down's syndrome there is a single large chromosome which corresponds to the long arm of chromosome 21 attached to the long arm of another chromosome (commonly chromosome 14). This translocation chromosome can be seen in chromosome spreads. Translocation Down's affected patients have only 46 chromosomes not the 47 found in the commoner form of Down's syndrome. Translocation Down's shows a familial pattern of inheritance with the presence of carriers who are themselves unaffected by Down's syndrome but who have an increased chance of passing it to their children. Translocation Down's syndrome is independent of maternal age.

9. A pericentric inversion occurs when there is an inverted piece of chromosome which includes the centromere. The inversion is symptomless until meiosis occurs when it can result in the death of the cells if a crossover occurs in the inverted region.

10. *In situ* hybridization is achieved by first separating the strands of DNA by high temperature melting. Labelled DNA probe (e.g. biotin labelled DNA) is then added and the conditions are adjusted to give annealing of the DNA. The labelled probe can hybridize with the cell's own DNA if the two sequences match. The label can then be visualized (e.g. using avidin and an enzyme). *In situ* hybridization can be used to identify and locate specific DNA sequences inside cells, e.g. it can be used to identify which cells are infected with a virus.

Chapter 14

1. Specimens for microbiology are living bacteria which allow cultures to be grown, and using these cultures biochemical and sensitivity tests can be carried out. The paraffin wax sections only contain dead cells which limits the investigation to staining and serology. The cultural and biochemical tests are more flexible and can identify a wider range of organisms.
2. Staining methods e.g. Gram can be used to identify the organism as Gram positive or negative. Immunological methods or *in situ* hybridization can be used to confirm the type of bacteria. Careful observation of the morphological changes in the tissue may help to identify the causative organisms.
3. Viruses (e.g. herpes), bacteria (e.g. *Staphylococcus aureus*), fungi (e.g. *Aspergillus fumigatus*) and protozoa (e.g. *Entamoeba histolytica*) can all appear in sections.
4. Amyloid is an abnormal protein which has the β-pleated sheet conformation that accumulates in certain pathological conditions. Amyloid is resistant to most proteolytic enzymes because of the unusual β-pleated sheet conformation.
5.

Amyloid type	Diseases which the amyloid is associated with
AL Amyloid light chain immune-associated amyloid	Multiple myeloma, Waldenstrom's disease
AA Reactive amyloid	Rheumatoid arthritis, TB, Hodgkin's disease, Familial Mediterranean fever
AE Endocrine related amyloid	Insulinomas, medullary carcinoma of thyroid
β-Amyloid	Alzheimer's disease, old age (80+)
AS Senile amyloid	
AF Familial amyloid	Familial amyloidosis

AD	Lichen amyloidosis
Dermal amyloid	
AH	Renal failure with haemodialysis
Haemodialysis associated amyloid	

6. (i) Congo red. (ii) Thioflavine. (iii) Methyl violet metachromasia. Congo red is the most useful as it can be used as a simple stain (staining amyloid a pink/red colour) in combination with polarization microscopy (amyloid shows a green birefringence) and as a fluorochrome. Thioflavine may be more sensitive but less selective and methyl violet is dependent on the batch of stain and is therefore less reliable.

Chapter 15

1. The numerical aperture is related to the resolving power of the lens which is one of the most important characteristics of any microscope lens. Numerical aperture is also related to the depth of field of the lens and determines how much depth of specimen is in focus at any one time.
2. Empty magnification is where the image is enlarged to give a bigger image but with no increase in detail. Empty magnification may even result in less detail being observable than at a lower but useful magnification. The useful magnification limit is approximately 1000 times the numerical aperture of the objective.
3. An achromatic lens is a lens that is partially corrected for chromatic aberration. The colour fringing (a spectrum of light produced by the lens) is greatly reduced but not totally eliminated.
4. The darkground microscope uses oblique illumination in the form of a hollow cone of light. None of the direct light can enter the objective so the field of view appears dark. Objects which can bend the light by diffraction or refraction will appear bright against this dark background.
5. In the polarizing microscope two polarizing filters are used with the first filter between the light source and the specimen and the second between the specimen and the eye. The first filter produduces plane polarized light and the second polarizing filter is rotated or 'crossed' so that in the absence of a specimen there is no direct illumination seen. Urea crystals are birefringent and rotate the plane of polarization allowing some light to pass through the second polarizing filter and so the crystals appear bright against a dark background.
6. Two filters are used in a conventional fluorescent microscope. The first filter is placed between the light source and the specimen and this allows only short wavelength light to pass. The second filter is placed between the specimen and the eye and

allows only long wavelength light to pass. Only fluorescent light which has been emitted by the specimen will be seen with this arrangement.

7. The human eye can be fooled by optical illusions and apparent size is a subjective assessment by the eye and the brain and not an absolute measurement.

8. 0.55 or 55% (area proportion is 110/200 = 0.55).

9. The density is not necessarily homogeneous. The amount of light passing through the lightly stained areas will be disproportionate to the amount of light coming through the darker areas and the amount of material will be underestimated.

Chapter 16

1. The conventional transmission electron microscope differs from the light microscope by using electrons instead of light, it has a better resolving ability since electrons can have much shorter wavelengths than light. The lenses in the EM are electromagnetic not glass, and magnification is changed by altering the magnetic strength of the lens rather than changing lenses as in the LM. The EM must work in a vacuum and this prevents looking at living specimens. The EM needs thinner sections and they need better support than in the LM and specimens are mounted on copper grids not glass slides. The image cannot be viewed directly in the EM but must use either a phosphorescent screen or taking a photograph. The image in the EM is always monochrome whilst the LM can be multicoloured. Contrast is achieved in the EM using heavy metal salts not the dyes used in LM.

2. Resin or plastic embedding is needed to give better support to the specimen and allow thinner sections to be cut. The plastics are also more stable than wax when subjected to a high vacuum and an electron beam and so they support the tissue better during examination.

3. There are no lenses used in the SEM to actually image the specimen so there are no lens aberrations. The condenser lenses used to focus the electron beam on to the specimen play no direct part in producing the image.

4. Critical point drying is the use of a liquid which has a critical temperature and pressure at which there is no distinction between the gaseous phase and the liquid phase. At this critical point the gas and liquid have exactly the same density. One such liquid is carbon dioxide. By dehydrating the tissues and then replacing the water with liquid carbon dioxide it is possible to remove the carbon dioxide without evaporation by simply warming it to above its critical temperature. The liquid becomes a gas without boiling or evaporating and can be allowed to escape gently without damaging the tissue.

5. It is necessary to coat SEM specimens to make them electrically conductive and gold is the best metal for this purpose. The electrical conductivity is needed to earth any static electrical charge which would otherwise interfere with the image.

6. The positive identification of a material in the light microscope is easier because there are a wide range of dyes which can be quite selective in their staining and dyes have a wide range of contrasting colours. In the EM there are only a few heavy metal ions available for use, they are less selective in their staining properties and will react with a wider range of materials. Finally the image is only in shades of grey so there is less distinction between materials.

7. The X-rays produced in the EM will have wavelengths characteristic of the elements within the specimen so by examining the spectrum of the X-rays it is possible to determine which elements are present in the specimen.

Index